Self-Assessment Colour Review of

Veterinary Cytology

Dog, Cat, Horse and Cow

Kathleen P Freeman

DVM BS MS PhD DipECVCP MRCVS
Killin, Perthshire, UK

MANSON PUBLISHING/TH

Acknowledgements

My sincere thanks to Joan Duncan for helping with this book. She has been a source of inspiration and motivation. Her attention to detail and willingness to help a friend and colleague is much appreciated.

Picture acknowledgements

29b and 137b courtesy of Heather Holloway
48a courtesy of Elizabeth Welsh

Copyright © 2007 Manson Publishing Ltd
ISBN: 978-1-84076-071-2

A CIP catalogue record for this book is available from the British Library.

For full details of all Manson Publishing Ltd titles please write to:
Manson Publishing Ltd, 73 Corringham Road, London NW11 7DL, UK.
Tel: +44(0)20 8905 5150
Fax: +44(0)20 8201 9233
Email: manson@mansonpublishing.com
Website: www.mansonpublishing.com

Commissioning editor: Jill Northcott
Project manager: Paul Bennett
Copy editor: Peter Beynon
Design and layout: Cathy Martin, Presspack Computing Ltd
Colour reproduction: Tenon & Polert Colour Scanning Ltd, Hong Kong
Printed by: New Era Printing Company Ltd, Hong Kong

Preface

This book aims to provide a representative sample of cytology cases encountered in a variety of diagnostic situations. It is not an inclusive text covering all conditions but offers a variety of cytology features and patterns from which anyone interested in veterinary cytology can continue to learn and test their knowledge. Bone marrow is covered by only a very few cases, since readers should not be misled and believe that they might be able to interpret a bone marrow from a single cytological field – they also need extensive knowledge and experience in haematology.

The format throughout the text encourages description and interpretation of the cytological specimens represented in the photomicrographs. The exercise of description is one that should not be ignored and, laborious as it may seem to those making their first attempts, it is critical for the development of a discriminating cytologist. The process of description provides a guide to a systematic method for covering the cellular and noncellular material that is present.

It is important to admit when cells or features are recognized but cannot be categorized. Knowledge of the range of 'normal' for various sites and types of specimens is critical. The recognition of normality provides the basis for recognition of deviations from 'normal' and the presence of disease. It is vitally important that the student of cytology strives to obtain and examine a variety of specimens that represent 'normal' for the age, system, physiological status, species, method of collection, method of cytological presentation and staining. Only by an appreciation of the range of presentations that can represent a 'normal' collection can one become comfortable with the various types of specimens and their interpretation.

The process of description itself is often helpful in arriving at a suitable interpretation. By taking time to describe, the mental process of discriminating between various broad categories of pathology and the more specific conditions that may occur at a particular site or with a particular species becomes a systematic process of inclusion or elimination.

Once the student of cytology becomes comfortable with the descriptive process, the ability to provide an interpretation, taking into account the description of the smear and the clinical history, also requires practice. One of the most common mistakes is to let the clinical history dictate the interpretation of the cytological specimen. The clinical history should provide a background from which interpretation should take some clues. One or several conditions or processes may be possible given a particular history, but there must also be strong cytological evidence for a particular interpretation before it can be given.

The degree of confidence that one has in the interpretation is also important. This may vary with experience and with the degree of clarity and correlation between the cytological specimen and the clinical history. The degree of certainty of the reporting cytologist is of crucial importance to the clinician, who can then balance the clinical appearance and history against the cytological description and interpretation to help determine a clinical or working diagnosis.

So, to those readers who wish to embark upon the journey of cytological exploration, I urge you to continue to strive to be true to the classic exercises of description and interpretation. Seek histological and/or clinical follow-up where and when it is appropriate. Continue to learn the fascinating science and art of cytological diagnosis!

Kathleen P Freeman

Contributors

A Rick Alleman DVM PhD DipACVP DipABVP
College of Veterinary Medicine, University of Florida, Gainesville, Florida, USA

Joan Duncan BVMS PhD DipRCPath CertVR MRCVS
NationWide Laboratories, Poulton-le-Fylde, Lancashire, UK

Corinne Fournel-Fleury DVM PhD DipECVCP HDR
Ecole Nationale Veterinaire de Lyon, Marcy L'Etoile, France

Kathleen P Freeman DVM BS MS PhD DipECVCP MRCVS
Killin, Perthshire, UK

Karen L Gerber BVSc (Pretoria) BVSc (Hons) DipACVP MRCVS
Axiom Veterinary Laboratories, Newton Abbot, Devon, UK

J Michael Harter DVM
Animal Medical Clinic, Rockford, Illinois, USA

Heather Holloway MA VetMB CertVC DipRCPath MRCVS
Idexx Laboratories, Wetherby, West Yorkshire, UK

Hugh Larkin MVB PhD MRCPath MECVCP MRCVS
School of Veterinary Medicine, St George's University, Grenada, West Indies

Sally Lester DVM MVSc DipACVP
Central Laboratory for Veterinarians, Langley, British Columbia, Canada

Kostas Papasouliotis DVM PhD DipRCPath DipECVCP MRCVS
School of Veterinary Science, University of Bristol, Langford, UK

Anne Lanevschi-Pietersma DVM MS DipACVP ECVCP
Apartado 23, A Estrada 36680 Spain

Mark D G Pinches BVSc MSc MRCVS
School of Veterinary Science, University of Bristol, Langford, UK

Shashi K Ramaiah DVM PhD DACVP DABT
College of Veterinary Medicine and Biomedical Sciences, Texas A and M University, College Station, Texas, USA

Federico Sacchini MVB DipSCPCA MPhil MRCVS
Idexx Laboratories, Wetherby, West Yorkshire, UK

Elizabeth Villiers BVSc DECVCP DipRCPath CertSAM CertVR MRCVS
University of Cambridge, Cambridge, UK

Abbreviations

ACTH	adrenocorticotrophic hormone	FIP	feline infectious peritonitis
AIDS	acquired immune deficiency syndrome	FIV	feline immunodeficiency virus
		FNA	fine needle aspirate
ALP	alkaline phosphatase	GM-CSF	granulocyte macrophage-colony stimulating factor
ALT	alanine aminotransferase	H&E	haematoxylin and eosin (stain)
APTT	activated partial prothrombin time	HDDS	high-dose dexamethasone suppression (test)
AST	aspartate aminotransferase	LDDS	low-dose dexamethasone suppression (test)
ASVCP	American Society for Veterinary Clinical Pathology	NADPH	nicotinamide adenine dinucleotide phosphate
BIN	bronchial intraepithelial neoplasia	NASDA	napthol ASD-acetate (esterase)
BUN	blood urea nitrogen	NCC	nucleated cell count
CBC	complete blood count	PAS	periodic acid-Schiff (stain)
CBP	centroblastic polymorphic	PCR	polymerase chain reaction
CFU	colony forming unit	PCV	packed cell volume
CNS	central nervous system	PEG	percutaneous endoscopically-guided gastrotomy (tubes)
CSF	cerebrospinal fluid		
DLH	domestic longhaired (cat)	PT	prothrombin time
DSH	domestic shorthaired (cat)	RBC	red blood cell
EDTA	ethylenediamine tetra-acetic acid	SAA	serum amyloid A (protein)
		SCC	squamous cell carcinoma
EGC	eosinophilic granuloma complex	SG	specific gravity
		TP	total protein
ELISA	enzyme-linked immunoabsorbent assay	V-BTA	veterinary bladder tumour antigen (test)
FeLV	feline leukaemia virus	WBC	white blood cell

Conversion factors

	SI units	Conversion factor	Old units
Haematology			
PCV	l/l	100	%
RBCs	$\times 10^{12}$/l	1	$\times 10^{6}$/l
Erytrocytes	$\times 10^{9}$/l	1	$\times 10^{3}$/l
Nucleated cell count	$\times 10^{9}$/l	1	$\times 10^{3}$/μl
Eosinophils	$\times 10^{9}$/l	1	$\times 10^{3}$/l
Biochemistry			
ACTH	ng/ml	1	pg/ml
Albumin	g/l	0.1	g/dl
Bilirubin	μmol/l	0.059	mg/dl
Cholesterol	mmol/l	38.61	mg/dl
Cortisol	nmol/l	0.036	μg/dl
Globulin	g/l	0.1	g/dl
Glucose	mmol/l	18	mg/dl
Total protein	g/l	10	g/dl
Total thyroxine (T4)	nmol/l	0.0777	μg/dl
Triglyceride	mmol/l	88.6	mg/dl
Urea nitrogen	mmol/l	2.8	mg/dl

Classification of cases

Cardiorespiratory system
4, 11, 13, 15, 20, 25, 27, 32, 37, 49, 51,
65, 73, 79, 80, 85, 99, 118, 145, 148,
159, 161

Ear, nose and throat
5, 6, 17, 54, 61, 63, 69, 117, 139, 142,
146, 152, 153, 159

Fluid classification
3, 68, 102

Gastrointestinal system
30, 39, 48, 50, 67, 76, 83, 110, 123,
128, 138, 143, 160

General interpretation
2, 12, 52, 70, 78, 82, 84, 93, 96, 100,
105, 112, 122, 125, 129, 133, 134, 144,
158, 165,

Infections
9, 18, 33, 42, 95, 97, 124, 164

Liver
10, 29, 41, 66, 72, 92, 108, 113, 119

Lymphatic system
21, 36, 45

Mammary glands
98, 120

Methodology
56, 58, 74, 107, 111, 131

Musculoskeletal system
1, 43, 86, 150, 154, 155, 163,

Neoplasia
7, 14, 22, 23, 26, 31, 34, 40, 46, 47, 53,
55, 60, 64, 71, 77, 81, 87, 90, 101, 104,
109, 115, 126, 127, 136, 140, 149, 157,
162

Reproductive system
8, 35, 38, 94, 121, 135, 141, 147

Skin
16, 19, 24, 28, 44, 57, 75, 88, 89, 91,
103, 106, 116, 130, 132, 151, 156

Urogenital system
59, 62, 114, 137

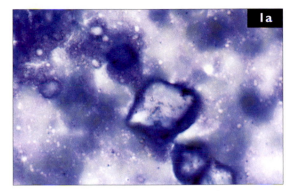

1 An 18-month-old German Shepherd Dog-cross presented with a dome-shaped mass of approximately 3 cm diameter in the area of the right distal antebrachium, near the elbow joint. Gritty chalky material with a cheesy consistency was aspirated and a smear prepared.
a What can be seen in the smear (**1a**) (Wright–Giemsa, ×100 oil)?
b What is your diagnosis?

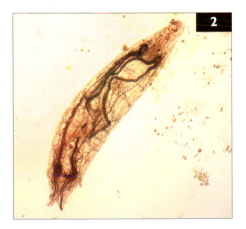

2 A five-year-old female Yorkshire Terrier presented with a two-day history of colitis-like diarrhoea. The owner brought in a faecal sample she had picked up within minutes of the dog defecating.
a What is the organism shown (**2**) (unstained saline wet mount, ×100 oil)?
b How can this appear in minutes?

1 a Refractile crystalline material of various sizes. In other fields (not illustrated) there are a few spindle cells and macrophages. A few multinucleated macrophages are also present.

b Calcinosis circumscripta (also called calcium gout, apocrine cystic calcinosis or tumoral calcinosis). This condition is considered to be a subcategory of calcinosis cutis. Its aetiopathogenesis is poorly understood. It occurs primarily in young, large-breed dogs and a predisposition in German Shepherd Dogs has been identified. It has been reported in the cervical spine, with spinal cord compression, the tongue and the skin, particularly on the extremities, adjacent to joints, and over pressure points. Boxers and Boston Terriers may be predisposed to lesions at the base of the pinna and on the cheek.

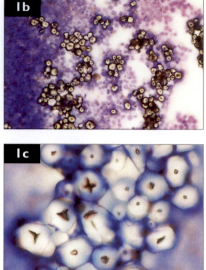

The lesions are usually single but some cases have multiple or bilaterally symmetrical lesions. The amount of crystalline material and associated granulomatous and fibroplastic response may vary amongst individuals; however, abundant crystalline material is usually present, as shown in this case. The radiographic and histological appearance are also characteristic. Treatment is by surgical removal and lesions have not been reported to recur following surgery.

In humans, calcinosis circumscripta has been associated with hyperphosphataemic imbalance and is considered to be familial. It has not been determined whether such an imbalance may play a role in some cases of calcinosis circumscripta in dogs.

The irregular crystalline material obtained from aspirates of foci of calcinosis circumscripta must not be confused with the starch crystals that are contaminants from powdered gloves (**1b, c**) (Wright–Giemsa, ×25 and ×100 oil, respectively). Starch crystals are small and oval to angular. At high magnification a characteristic central cross, slit or oval structure can be seen. Glove powder is a frequent contaminant of cytological specimens collected when gloves are worn or in an area where powdered gloves are used. When found in a body cavity fluid specimen with granulomatous inflammation or history of a mass, the possibility of a talc-associated granuloma from previous contamination with glove powder should be considered.

2 a A larva of a dipteran fly – a maggot. It is a pseudoparasite. The breathing spiracles can be seen on the bottom left.

b Some flies are viviparous, depositing live larvae (rather than eggs) on fresh faeces.

3 A 12-year-old Thoroughbred-cross gelding presented with a history of chronic weight loss. He had a poor coat and was emaciated at the time of referral. A peritoneal fluid specimen was submitted for body fluid analysis and cytological evaluation. Analysis revealed: erythrocyte count = $20 \times 10^9/l$; NCC = $15 \times 10^9/l$; TP = 32 g/l. The reference intervals for equine (and bovine) pleural and abdominal fluid are shown.

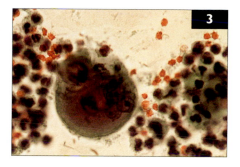

a How would you classify this fluid?
b What cell types can be seen in this photomicrograph (3) (Papanicolaou, ×100 oil)?
c What is your diagnosis?

Category	TP	NCC
Transudate	<15 g/l	<5 × 10⁹/l
Modified transudate	5–35 g/l	<15 × 10⁹/l
Exudate	>35 g/l	>10 × 10⁹/l

4 A 15-month-old entire male English Springer Spaniel presented with a chronic, worsening productive cough. The dog had shown no response to a one-week course of doxycycline and it had recently become anorexic. On clinical examination the dog was slightly pyrexic. Radiographs of the thorax revealed a bronchopneumonia and endoscopy a severe tonsillitis, laryngitis and tracheitis. A smear of some expectorated material was made.

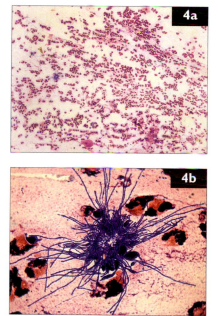

a Describe the features illustrated (4a, b) (modified Wright's, ×10 and ×100 respectively).
b What is your interpretation of these findings?
c Which treatments are most efficacious for this organism?
d What other conditions is this organism associated with?

3 a Modified transudate.
b A few erythrocytes and many neutrophils. In the centre of the field, there are two cells with features of malignancy. One is small and mononucleated and the other is large and contains multiple nuclei, several of which are not in the plane of focus. The nuclei often contain uneven nuclear membrane thickening and distinct nucleoli. The cytoplasm has a crisply defined border and central dense character, with a more delicate periphery of endoplasmic and ectoplasmic differentiation, which is consistent with squamous differentiation.
c Squamous cell carcinoma (SCC) of the stomach. The neutrophilic response is characteristic for this type of tumour. Squamous cells are found in peritoneal fluid when the tumour has caused rupture or ulceration of the stomach wall and communication with the peritoneal cavity, or when there has been lymphatic metastasis, often with ulceration or rupture of lymphatics that allows cells into the peritoneal cavity. Therefore, cancer cells may not be apparent in all cases with gastric SCC and their detection will depend on the stage of the disease, its progression and the number of cells shed into the peritoneal cavity. Cancer cells may fail to be represented in smears or may be missed or masked by inflammation or haemorrhage if present only in small numbers.

SCC of the stomach in the horse has a poor prognosis since it is often not diagnosed until advanced disease and/or metastasis is present. Endoscopic evaluation is often helpful in the diagnosis of oesophageal or gastric SCC, particularly if cancer cells are not apparent in the peritoneal fluid. Washings of the stomach or brushings of suspicious lesions have also been used successfully in the diagnosis of gastric SCC in the horse when peritoneal fluid was not rewarding in demonstrating cancer cells.

4 a The low-power photomicrograph indicates a very highly cellular sample with large numbers of neutrophils contained within copious amounts of mucinous material. Many of the neutrophils are degenerate and smeared. Within this mix are a number of basophilic 'fluffy' particles. The high-power photomicrograph shows one of the fluffy particles in greater detail. The particle is composed of numerous basophilic filamentous rod-shaped organisms, whose terminal portions in some cases have become club shaped. The neutrophils present show karyorhexis and karyolysis.
b These findings indicate a severe septic neutrophilic inflammation. The organisms have the typical appearance of *Actinomyces* species in their 'ray fungi' form as seen in actinomycosis. The clubbed ends are gelatinous sheaths containing deposits of calcium phosphate.
c Prolonged antibiotic therapy with penicillin, amoxycillin, chloramphenicol and clindamycin is the most efficacious treatment.
d *Actinomyces* species are gram-positive, microaerophilic to anaerobic, non-acid-fast rods that show occasional branching. They are usually commensals of the oropharynx and are associated with pneumonia, pyothorax, subcutaneous infections and septic arthritis.

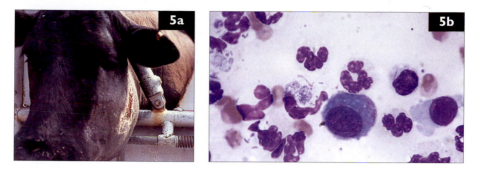

5 A firm ulcerated mass is noted on the jaw of a Friesian cow (5a). An FNA is collected and a smear made (5b) (Wright–Giemsa, ×100 oil).
a What cells are present?
b What is your diagnosis?

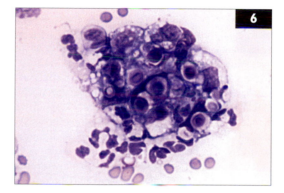

6 A three-year-old neutered male DSH cat presents with inspiratory dyspnoea and severe nasal congestion of four months' duration. The cat has lost weight and shown partial anorexia in the last few weeks. Physical examination reveals approximately 10% dehydration, hyperthermia (39.8°C [103.6°F]), unilateral mucosanguineous nasal discharge and ipsilateral submandibular lymph node enlargement. The referring veterinarian had administered enrofloxacin, doxycycline, and amoxicillin/clavulanic acid successively and no improvement was noted. The vaccinations are up-to-date and the cat is free roaming. A smear is prepared from the nasal discharge (6) (Wright's, ×100 oil).
a What is your diagnosis based on cytological observation?
b What other diagnostic tests can be performed to support this diagnosis?
c What treatment can be recommended?

5 a There is a mixed population of cells, including neutrophils, reactive macrophages and lymphocytes. There are also beaded, filamentous organisms.
b The cytological interpretation is subacute inflammation and infection; the organisms are consistent with *Actinobacillus* species.

6 a The cytological findings are consistent with neutrophilic infection and intralesional *Cryptococcus neoformans* microorganisms.
b Fungal culture can enable isolation and identification of the microorganisms if they are not found following cytological examination of a case in which *Cryptococcus* infection is suspected, or if confirmation of a diagnosis is needed. Antigen detection using serum, urine or CSF can be carried out to establish a diagnosis or for therapeutic monitoring: a titre as low as 1:1 is considered a positive test and diagnostic of cryptococcosis.
c Oral fluconazole and itraconazole are the preferred antimycotic drugs; ketoconazole is less effective and is associated with greater toxicity in cats. Treatment should be continued for four weeks following resolution of clinical signs or following a 100-fold decrease in titre levels, or until a negative post-treatment titre is obtained. The prognosis is better when respiratory or cutaneous lesions are involved (53% and 82%, respectively, of such cases are responsive to treatment) whereas the prognosis is guarded in cases where there is CNS or ocular involvement or if there is underlying FeLV or FIV infection. It is recommended to test the patient for FeLV and FIV prior to initiating therapy. This cat recovered following ten weeks of antimycotic therapy, and no recurrence was noted in a one-year follow-up examination.

Cryptococcus infection and organisms may be seen in a variety of types of specimens, but in cats they are most commonly found in CSF or nasal specimens. They may be seen in cutaneous lesions or in pericardial, abdominal or thoracic fluid, lymph node aspirates, respiratory cytology specimens or other sites, depending on whether the infection is localized or generalized and the presenting signs and avenues of investigation.

Cryptococcus organisms may be confused with tissue cells since the central organism may resemble a nucleus and the surrounding halo or capsule may be mistaken for boundaries of cytoplasm. In some cases the organisms may be refractile and be confused with particles of glove powder, which may also be refractile. Sometimes, cryptococcal organisms are small and may not have a prominent capsule; these may be difficult to distinguish from lysed erythrocytes or air bubbles if present only in small numbers. The organisms may display a wide range of diameters (from 5 to 20 microns). Accompanying inflammation may vary from slight to absent or granulomatous. An apparent absence of inflammation cannot be relied on to rule out infection.

Ultrastructurally, it has been shown that the capsule is formed by intertwined microfibrils radiating from the surface of the organism. A Mucicarmine or PAS stain will stain the surrounding capsule red or pink because of the mucopolysaccharide contents. The thickness of the capsule is believed to be related to the age and degree of degeneration of the organism, with younger, more well preserved elements showing less capsule. When budding is recognized, *Cryptococcus* will exhibit narrow-based budding.

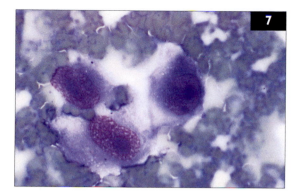

7 An eight-year-old Irish Setter presented with a mass in the right flank. An FNA was collected and a smear prepared.
a What cell types and features are present in this photomicrograph (7) (Wright–Giemsa, ×100 oil)?
b What is your diagnosis?

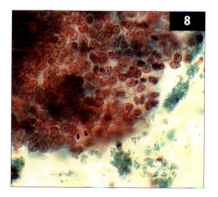

8 A six-year-old Thoroughbred broodmare presented with a history of repeated uterine infections that had been treated with repeated antibiotic infusions by indwelling catheter. The last treatment was given earlier in the day and the catheter was removed following collection of a uterine washing.
a What features are illustrated in this smear (8) (Papanicolaou, ×100 oil)?
b What is your interpretation of these findings?

7 a Many erythrocytes and several cells with features of malignancy. These cells have large, round to oval nuclei with coarsely clumped chromatin and large, round to oval nucleoli. The cytoplasm is moderate and wispy to fusiform, with poorly defined borders. The rest of the smear had a similar appearance, with a few to a moderate number of cells with similar features.

b Sarcoma. The features are not specific as to the type of sarcoma but the cytological features are considered to reflect an aggressive malignancy. The bloody nature of the aspirate may be due to contamination with blood, but the possibility of haemangiosarcoma should be considered when mesenchymal cells with features of malignancy are present. Evaluation for metastasis did not reveal any suspicious areas, so surgical removal was attempted. The histological diagnosis was haemangiosarcoma.

8 a There is some granular background precipitate that stains blue-green, and in the upper left corner of the figure there is a large, cohesive group of epithelial cells. These cells have large, oval nuclei, often containing clear chromatin and a single, distinct, central nucleolus. The cytoplasm is substantial. There is a single mitotic figure at the lower edge of the group. No inflammatory cells are visible.

b The cytological features are consistent with reactive epithelium associated with irritation from the treatment. This most likely represents damaged epithelium that is attempting to heal (with mitoses). It is within expected limits following treatment using an indwelling catheter. These features should not be mistaken for adenocarcinoma, although some of the cellular features may mimic adenocarcinoma.

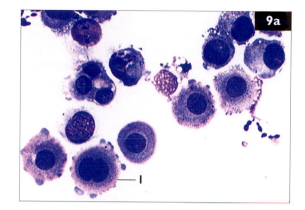

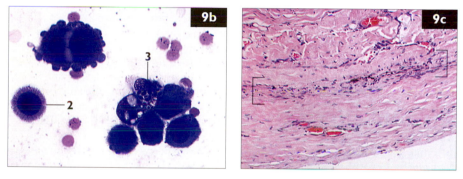

9 Pleural fluid was obtained from a 12-year-old neutered male Golden Retriever with clinical signs of dyspnoea and restrictive pericarditis on ultrasound and radiography. Smears were prepared from sediment from the fluid (9a, b) (both Wright–Giemsa, ×50 oil).

a The laboratory data and a cytological review indicated that the fluid was a modified transudate, with evidence of previous haemorrhage and a 'potential' underlying aetiology. What are the structures labelled 1, 2 and 3?

b Which special stains would you request on the cytology specimen to help confirm that the structures are yeast?

c List five more common types of fungal infections that can be isolated/identified in pleural fluid.

d A pericardectomy was performed a few days post cytology, and the pericardium was evaluated histologically. Identify the most significant pathological change (bracketed) (9c) (H&E, ×100 oil).

9 a 1 = reactive mesothelial cell, frequently binucleate (do not mistake these for neoplastic cells). **2** = reactive mesothelial cell with characteristic corona (peripheral frill), which is an artefact of slow drying and of no diagnostic significance. **3** = macrophage and/or reactive mesothelial cell with broad-based budding yeast-like structures, roughly 0.5 microns in length. The precise identification of the yeast-like organism was not obtained because the organism failed to grow on culture.

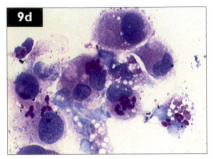

b (1) PAS. The dark pink or magenta structures seen in **9d** (PAS, ×100) are yeast within the cytoplasm of the macrophages. The nuclei are counterstained with haematoxylin. The glycoprotein in yeast stains magenta, therefore yeast is PAS-positive. (2) Silver stains can be used to stain fungal elements and yeast.

c *Histoplasma capsulatum*: dimorphic fungus (dogs, cats); *Cryptococcus neoformans*: encapsulated yeast, monomorphic organisms (dogs, cats); *Coccidioides immitis*: geophilic dimorphic fungus (dogs); *Blastomyces dermatitidis*: dimorphic fungus (dogs, cats); *Pneumocystis carinii*: fungal organism (dogs – bronchoalveolar lavage and lung).

d The parietal aspect of the pericardium shows subacute inflammation, characterized by congestion, oedema and a mild to moderate infiltrate of neutrophils and macrophages (at higher magnification and in other areas, segmental necrotizing vasculitis is recognizable).

Note: This case presents the opportunity to consider differential diagnoses for fungal infection. Of particular note is *Pneumocystis carinii*. Some older references refer to *P. carinii* as a protozoal organism. It has recently been reclassified as a fungus due to the DNA sequence of its 16S RNA subunit and the fact that its cell wall and intracellular organelles more closely resemble those of fungi.

P. carinii with pulmonary infection has been diagnosed in humans in premature or debilitated infants, patients with immunological disorders and immunoglobulin defects and in individuals treated with corticosteroids and chemotherapy. It has been found in high frequency in renal allograft patients and as a complication of AIDS. Since many of the conditions, treatments or corresponding disorders are present in animals, it may be more common in veterinary patients than previously realized. Although uncommon, extrapulmonary infections have been observed in immunocompromised humans with AIDS and it has been reported in pleural and peritoneal fluids. It may pass unnoticed in a cytological preparation unless the cytologist is aware of its characteristic appearance as extracellular amorphous, foamy material with a suggestion of small superimposed circlets. Such material may be present as 'casts' of alveoli with masses or organisms surrounded by a smooth border created by the boundaries of the alveolar wall. Only a few organisms may be within macrophages or neutrophils.

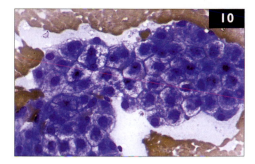

10 A six-year-old female Schnauzer presented with polyuria/polydipsia and frequent nocturnal urination. Physical examination revealed that the dog was bright and alert, slightly overweight and had a distended abdomen. An enlarged liver was evident on abdominal palpation. The rest of the physical examination was within normal limits. Abnormal biochemistry values were as follows: AST = 253 U/l (ref. = 14–38 U/l); ALT = 450 U/l (ref. = 10–71 U/l); ALP = 2,300 U/l (ref. = 4–110 U/l); glucose = 7.78 mmol/l (ref. = 4.4–7.0 mmol/l); bilirubin = 1.7 μmol/l (ref. = 0–6.8 μmol/l).

a Describe the cytological features seen in the FNA of the liver (10) (Wright–Giemsa, ×25), and give a cytological interpretation.

b Briefly discuss the biochemical profile. How does it support your cytological findings?

c Discuss additional diagnostic tests to confirm the underlying disease process.

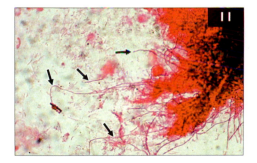

11 A ten-year-old spayed female barn cat presented with severe dyspnoea and cyanosis. Thoracocentesis yielded a foul-smelling, purulent, grey material. A smear of the material was made (11) (Gram's, ×100 oil).

a What are the structures arrowed?

b What are two organisms that have this kind of morphology?

c How can you differentiate between the two before culture results can be received?

10 a Clusters of well-differentiated hepatocytes are seen, most of which have indistinct cytoplasmic vacuolation. The cytoplasmic clearing caused by the vacuolation tends to be located in the periphery of the cell cytoplasm. The cytological interpretation is glycogen accumulation consistent with steroid hepatopathy.

b Elevated ALT and AST are suggestive of mild hepatic damage. The markedly elevated ALP without an increase in bilirubin is typical of steroid hepatopathy. This can be due to exogenous corticosteroid administration or endogenous corticosteroid release as seen in cases of Cushing's disease.

c A screening test such as the ACTH response test (very specific test with 85% sensitivity) can be used to confirm a diagnosis of Cushing's disease. In this case the basal cortisol concentration was 221 nmol/l (ref. = 25–260 nmol/l) and the post-ACTH concentration was 745 nmol/l (ref. = 260–660 nmol/l). This is strongly suggestive of Cushing's disease. Dogs with iatrogenic Cushing's disease usually have both basal and post-ACTH cortisol concentrations of <221 nmol/l. An LDDS test can also be used. An HDDS test is needed to differentiate between pituitary-dependent hyperadrenocorticism and adrenal tumour. HDD suppresses more than 50% of pituitary tumours. If HDD does not suppress, measurement of endogenous ACTH levels is needed (<20 ng/ml is consistent with an adrenal tumour, >50 ng/ml is supportive of pituitary-dependent hyperadrenocorticism; 20–50 ng/ml is 'grey zone' or nondiagnostic). Ultrasound evaluation of the adrenals may also be helpful.

Note: The interpretation of liver aspirate cytology is enhanced by knowledge of the clinical chemistry findings and endocrine testing, as illustrated in this case. Confidence in the interpretation of cytological findings and elimination of various differential diagnoses is dependent on provision of pertinent case information. If the cytological investigation is conducted before other studies, these features would indicate a need for additional investigation, and a chemistry profile and endocrine testing should be recommended.

Hepatocellular vacuolar change is also sometimes known as vacuolar hepatopathy or cytoplasmic rarefaction. It may be difficult to differentiate the 'fuzzy' vacuolation of glycogen accumulation and diffuse hydropic degeneration, while hepatic lipidosis is characterized by discrete, more crisply defined vacuoles. A PAS stain can be used to identify glycogen. Prior to diastase digestion, glycogen will stain bright pink with this stain. Following diastase digestion, glycogen will be removed and the pink staining reaction will be greatly decreased or absent.

11 a There is a clump of filamentous gram-negative rods.

b *Actinomyces* species and *Nocardia* species are bacterial genera that have this morphology. Of the two, *Actinomyces* is most likely in cases of pyothorax in the cat.

c An acid-fast stain (either Ziehl–Neelsen, or Kinyoun's Cold Acid-Fast [an easy one to do in-house]) would differentiate the two species; *Nocardia* species are partially acid-fast, whilst *Actinomyces* are acid-fast negative.

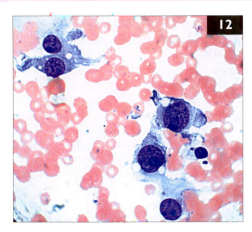

12 A seven-year-old neutered male Irish Setter presented with a subcutaneous/dermal lump on the flank that was dark red to red-black when shaved and aspirated.
a Describe the features of the cells seen in this smear prepared from the aspirate (12) (Wright–Giemsa, ×50 oil).
b What is your interpretation?

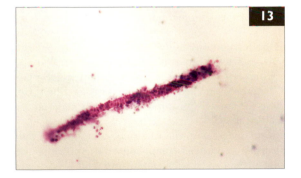

13 A 14-year-old carriage horse in New York City presented with a history of chronic coughing. A tracheal washing was collected and a smear prepared.
a What is the structure shown in this photomicrograph (13) (Alcian Blue-PAS overlaid on Papanicolaou, ×40)?
b What is its significance?

12 a There are a moderate number of erythrocytes in the background of the smear, with a few lymphocytes and neutrophils. There are multiple cells with features of malignancy. These have oval nuclei with prominent nucleoli. The cytoplasm is moderate and varies from ovoid to elongated or wispy, and it is moderately blue.
b The cytological features are consistent with malignancy, most likely of mesenchymal origin. Given the cytological appearance of mesenchymal malignancy, the pigmented macroscopic appearance, the location and the bloody background, haemangiosarcoma should be a primary consideration.

Haemangiosarcoma was confirmed on histological examination following surgical removal. Cutaneous haemangiosarcoma has the potential for metastasis and aggressive biological behaviour. Evaluation for possible metastases or multiple sites of involvement is recommended.

13 a An 'asbestos body'; the current preferred term is ferruginous body. These fibrillary structures have been associated with reaction to inhaled fibres of asbestos, but they may occur with inhalation of a number of different mineral fibres.
b The significance of finding a ferruginous body in a tracheal washing from a horse is uncertain, since they are rarely observed. In humans they are linked to the development of mesotheliomas and bronchogenic carcinoma. Large numbers of ferruginous bodies in broncholavage fluid from humans probably reflect occupational exposure, whereas occasional bodies are a nonspecific finding. All inhabitants of modern urban societies have ferruginous bodies in their lungs, but usually the concentration in members of the general population is so low that they are rarely found in routinely prepared sections of lung or in respiratory cytology specimens. A Perl's Prussian Blue stain may increase sensitivity in detection of ferruginous bodies, since they often contain iron and stain positively (blue).

The finding of the ferruginous body in this horse may have been linked to his urban environment and working conditions. It is included in this book as an illustration of the variety of features that can be found when a large case volume is seen. Differential diagnoses may include other types of fibres from environmental contamination. These are not easily confused with plant material, since plant material usually contains visible cell walls.

In order to become familiar with the variety of contaminants that frequently occur with equine respiratory specimens (plant material, spores, pollen), collection of material by shaking of hay over a collection pot and leaving a slide sitting on a window ledge for several hours is recommended. The material collected in this manner can be prepared and stained for routine evaluation and provide examples of elements that commonly occur as environmental contaminants. The types of contaminants may vary between stables, ventilation systems, different batches of hay, management styles and during various times of the year, so periodic evaluation of environmental contaminants is often useful for quality assurance and quality control with equine respiratory specimens.

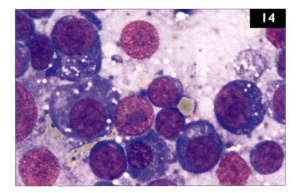

14 An FNA is collected from a canine lymph node.
a What cells are shown in this smear (14) (May–Grünwald–Giemsa, ×100 oil)?
b What is your diagnosis and what are the differential diagnoses?

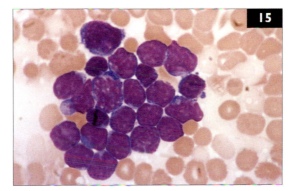

15 A nine-year-old three quarter-bred hunter was running badly. Excessive fluid was identified in the pleural space. A sample of fluid was withdrawn; it was light yellow and clear, and had an NCC of 5.5×10^9/l and a TP of 24 g/l. A cytospun smear of pleural fluid contained a mixed cell population including erythrocytes, neutrophils, macrophages and mesothelial cells, and many clusters of cells (15) (Wright–Giemsa, ×100 oil).
a How would you classify the fluid?
b What are the cells shown in 15?
c What is your diagnosis?

14 a A cluster of lymphoid cells at different stages, more or less arrested between immunoblasts and plasma cells.

b Diagnosis: immunoblastic, plasmablastic lymphoma (B-cell phenotype: CD79a+, CD3-, cIg+). This is probably a blastic transformation of a lymphoplasmacytic lymphoma (immunocytoma). Differential diagnosis: atypical immunoblastic hyperplasia, but the blockage at a plasmablastic stage suggests a lymphoma is more likely.

Note: The classification of various types of lymphomas histologically and cytologically, and the significance of these findings, are currently topics of intense investigation and scientific discussion. Several classification systems have been proposed, within which there is some variation in the types and terminology applied.

The application of various markers (e.g. CD79a, CD3– and cIg+, as used in this case) has enabled a better understanding of the cell lineage and level of differentiation from which various lymphomas and other types of cancer are derived. Other investigators are concentrating on the genetic alterations that may accompany these phenotypes and the treatments that may have an application based on these alterations.

To date, it has been recognized that lymphomas of B-cell origin generally have a better prognosis and response to treatment than those of T-cell origin. Some subtypes of lymphoma are known to have certain predispositions or common presentations. For example, T-cell lymphoblastic lymphomas are often accompanied by a mediastinal mass and paraneoplastic hypercalcaemia; centroblastic, medium-size cell macronucleolated subtype often presents in stage IV or stage V, so evaluation of internal organs and blood/bone marrow should be emphasized. However, it is not possible to predict accurately the clinical course and response to treatment in each individual animal. Perhaps in the future it may be feasible to more accurately tailor treatment and/or prognosis based on a combination of cytological morphology, panels of markers to help define the cell type of origin and genetic analyses to determine the underlying defect or combination of alterations that has resulted in the malignancy.

15 a The fluid is a modified transudate, as the NCC and TP values are within the ranges usually seen for this type of fluid.

b There is a mixed cell population. The cells are pleomorphic round cells showing anisocytosis and anisokaryosis. The large nuclei and thin rims of cytoplasm suggest they are of lymphoid origin. The cytoplasm is intensely basophilic. The nuclei have irregular borders and clumped chromatin, and nucleoli are present in some. The cells are considered to be neoplastic lymphocytes.

c Lymphosarcoma. The horse was euthanased and lymphosarcoma was confirmed on postmortem examination.

Note: Reference values for NCCs and classification of effusions in large animals differ from those for small animal specimens. (Guidelines for fluid classification in cows and horses are shown in question 3.)

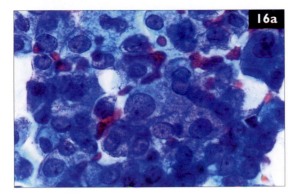

16 An FNA was collected from a cutaneous mass on a four-year-old Boxer (16a) (Diff-Quik, × 100 oil).
a Give a list of differential diagnoses.
b What further tests should be carried out?
c Summarize the major differences in prognoses between the differential diagnoses.

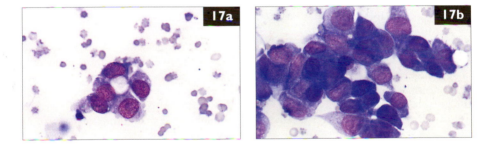

17 A 13-year-old cat was presented with a smooth nodular lesion in the external ear canal. Direct smears of the contents were made (17a, b) (Wright–Giemsa, ×40 and ×100 oil, respectively).
a Describe the cells present.
b What is the cell line of origin of these cells?
c Are there features present that suggest malignancy?

16 a The cytological features are consistent with a 'round cell tumour'. Major differentials are histiocytoma, mast cell tumour, lymphoma or transmissible venereal tumour.
b Stain with Wright–Giemsa initially. Although both Diff-Quik and Wright–Giemsa are Romanowsky stains, Diff-Quik may not stain the granules well or at all in some mast cell tumours. Other stains used to highlight the granules in mast

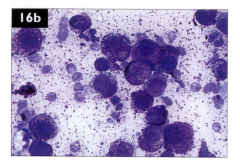

cells would include Toluidine Blue. In the photomicrograph provided (16a) a few faint granules are apparent in some cells on close inspection. 16b (Wright–Giemsa, ×100 oil) from the same lesion shows the granules of the mast cells clearly.
c It is important to identify mast cell tumours as they may lead to regional and widespread metastases. Systemic effects include gastric ulceration and/or systemic mastocytosis. They require prompt and wide surgical excision and careful handling, as degranulation during manipulation may lead to hypotension and shock. Histiocytomas, on the other hand, are usually benign and may regress spontaneously. Lymphoma carries a poor prognosis, although it may often respond to chemotherapy for a time. Transmissible venereal tumours may transfer between individuals. The prognosis is variable and cannot be predicted based on the cytological appearance.

17 a There is marked pleomorphism and anisokaryosis of the cells in 17b. The cells in 17a are arranged in an acinar or ductal configuration around a central lumen. Many cells have a high nuclear:cytoplasmic ratio, with a coarse nuclear chromatin pattern and prominent nucleoli. Some of these nucleoli are macronucleoli (>5μm diameter).
b The adherent nature of these cells indicates an epithelial origin. The nuclei in 17a are at the periphery of the cells, indicating an acinar or ductal formation, which, in turn, suggests a tumour of secretory or glandular tissue.
c Pleomorphism, anisokaryosis, increased nuclear:cytoplasmic ratio, a coarse chromatin pattern, macronucleoli and variation in nucleolar size and shape are all criteria of malignancy. Given the presence of these criteria, the probable glandular origin, and the site of the lesion, these features most likely reflect a ceruminous gland adenocarcinoma. Histological evaluation confirmed a ceruminous gland adenocarcinoma with lymphatic spread.
Note: Ceruminous gland tumours are more frequent in cats than in dogs. They are often associated with a history of chronic irritation and infection. Hyperplasia and adenomas may be difficult to differentiate cytologically and clinically. Adenocarcinomas are diagnosed based on features of malignancy. Adenocarcinomas are locally invasive and may metastasize to regional lymph nodes. Occasionally, more distant metastases are identified.

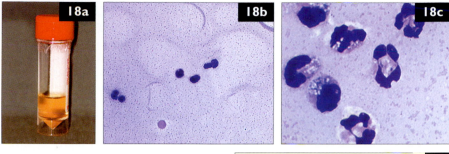

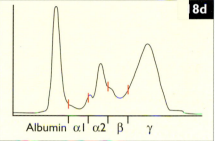

18 This straw-coloured ascitic fluid (18a) was obtained by abdominocentesis from a two-year-old cat with a history of pyrexia and abdominal distension.
a Classify the fluid using both the photo-micrographs (18b, c) (Wright–Giemsa, ×50 oil and ×100 oil, respectively) and the laboratory data (TP = 65.5 g/l; SG = 1.042; WBCs = 0.43 × 10^9/l; RBCs = 0.01 × 10^{12}/l).
b Given the high fluid protein concentration, electrophoresis was requested. Interpret the trace (18d).
c Although the electrophoresis pattern is not pathognomonic for specific conditions, in the context of the other findings in this particular case, what diagnosis should be at the top of the differential list?

19 A ten-year-old neutered male Rottweiler has a cutaneous mass on the 3rd digit of its left hind foot. The mass has been present for three weeks and is growing. The mass is dark red and the skin is hairless. An FNA is collected (19) (Giemsa, ×100 oil).
a Examine the nuclei – are there any criteria of malignancy?
b Examine the cytoplasm – are there granules present?
c What are the diagnosis and prognosis?
d What would you do next?

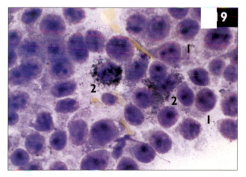

18 a Modified transudate (sometimes called 'low cell exudate'), a category combining both properties of transudates (NCC <1 × 10^9/l) and exudates (TP >30g/l). At low magnification, the background is finely granular with lighter staining crescent artefacts. This background suggests increased globular protein concentration (**18b**).

b Electrophoresis reveals (1) alpha-2 spike consistent with an acute phase response: proteins in the alpha-2 region are produced by the liver in response to a network of cytokines involved in inflammation; and (2) a marked polyclonal elevation of gamma globulins consistent with a polyclonal gammopathy. Overall, electrophoresis is consistent with a marked, established inflammatory process.

c Feline infectious peritonitis (FIP). A tentative clinical diagnosis of FIP is based on multiple strong positive results in a panel of tests: appropriate clinical signs (e.g. ascites; age [young]; fluid albumin:globulin ratio <0.8; high fluid and plasma globulin concentrations; electrophoresis (trace in this case is classic); positive coronavirus antibody on fluid or serum/plasma (this patient was FIP/coronavirus positive with a titre of 1:2560 [ELISA test]).

Note: A well-known adage regarding FIP is that it is a 'diagnosis of exclusion and support' when suggestive cytological findings are present. Other possible causes of effusion need to be excluded, while additional supporting evidence for FIP is needed. FIP is typically a disease of young (<2 years of age) or older cats. Hypergammaglobulinaemia is frequently present, as well as albumin:globulin ratios of <0.8 in serum and effusion fluids. Polyclonal gammopathies with similar protein electrophoresis findings in serum and peritoneal fluid are supportive. Lymphopenia is often present. A positive titre for feline coronavirus does not provide support for this diagnosis since many cats without disease will have positive titres. The level of antibody titre is not of diagnostic or prognostic significance. A negative titre in a healthy cat suggests that the cat has not been exposed to feline coronavirus. A negative titre in a sick cat does not rule out FIP since some cats with fulminant FIP may present with negative titres due to anergy or antigen-antibody complex formation that limits the ability to detect antibodies to this virus.

19 a The nuclei are quite large with stippled chromatin and many have prominent nucleoli. Some have a single, large, fairly central nucleolus. Others have two or multiple nucleoli (1). The nuclear:cytoplasmic ratio is increased.

b A few cells have dark green/black cytoplasmic granules – these are melanin granules (2).

c This is a melanoma. Given the site, paucity of melanin granules and the nuclear features, the tumour is malignant. These tumours often metastasize to local and distant sites, so the prognosis is guarded.

d Tumour staging is required before treatment. The local lymph node should be palpated and aspirated. Chest radiographs should be taken to rule out pulmonary metastasis. If there is no evidence of metastasis, the affected digit should be amputated.

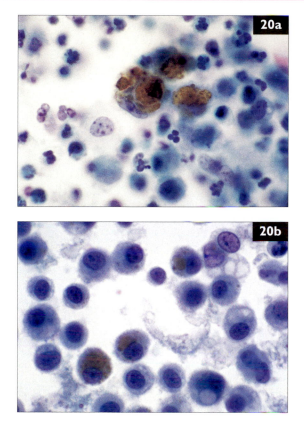

20 A three-year-old Thoroughbred racehorse is referred for investigation of poor performance. A bronchoalveolar lavage specimen is collected as part of the work up.

a What cell types are present in these photomicrographs (20a, b) (Papanicolaou, ×50 oil and ×100 oil)?

b What differences do you notice in the siderophages shown in these photomicrographs?

c What is your interpretation of the cytological findings?

20 a There are a few to a moderate number of neutrophils and a moderate number to many macrophages in **20a**. There are three siderophages (macrophages containing large clumps of green pigment) in the upper central portion of the figure. There is a small amount of thin mucus in the background, with many macrophages in **20b**. Three siderophages are present.

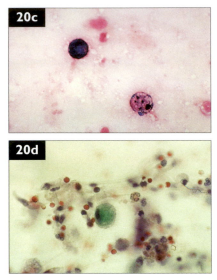

b The siderophages in **20a** contain larger, more darkly stained clumps of haemosiderin compared with the siderophages in **20b**. The siderophages in **20b** contain finer, more lightly stained granules of haemosiderin. The finer, more lightly stained siderophages have been designated as 'early siderophages' and usually occur between three and 14 days following blood instillation or observation of bleeding endoscopically. The siderophages containing larger, more darkly stained clumps of haemosiderin are termed 'aged siderophages' and are observed more than 14 days following blood instillation or endoscopic haemorrhage.

The ease with which haemosiderin is recognized in the Papanicolaou-stained smears is an advantage of this stain over Romanowsky stains for equine respiratory specimens. A Perl's Prussian Blue stain can be applied directly over the Papanicolaou-stained preparation if additional confirmation of the presence of iron is desired. **20c** (Perl's Prussian Blue, ×16) shows several macrophages in an equine tracheal washing with blue, granular cytoplasmic material confirmatory of iron and the presence of haemosiderin. **20d** (Perl's Prussian Blue, ×25) shows a diffusely stained, pale blue macrophage with some orange erythrocytes in the background of a tracheal washing. In some specimens these diffusely stained, iron-positive cells can be detected in cells without the presence of recognizable haemosiderin granules. Their significance is not certain but they are only consistently found in specimens from horses with confirmed pulmonary haemorrhage.

c The simultaneous appearance of 'early siderophages' and 'aged siderophages' in a respiratory cytology specimen supports the presence of haemorrhage on more than one occasion. Other features of the smear (not all of which are illustrated) include abundant thin mucus, many active macrophages, few to moderate number of neutrophils and focal and slight atypia of columnar and cuboidal epithelial cells consistent with bronchitis and bronchiolitis. No eosinophils were seen. This combination of cellular and noncellular features is consistent with the pattern of exercise-induced pulmonary haemorrhage.

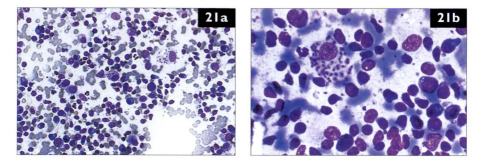

21 A five-year-old Boxer presented with acute onset of unilateral epistaxis. The dog appeared underweight and physical examination revealed generalized lymphadenopathy. An FNA was obtained from the left popliteal lymph node.
a The aspirate is moderately cellular with some blood contamination. Describe the main changes present in 21a (Wright–Giemsa, ×50 oil)? The large cell in the centre of 21b (Wright–Giemsa, ×100 oil) represents a mononuclear phagocyte. Describe the organisms within the cytoplasm? What is your diagnosis?
b Laboratory investigation revealed nonregenerative anaemia, hyperglobulinaemia characterized by polyclonal gammopathy and mild renal azotaemia. A coagulation panel was normal. How can the epistaxis be explained?

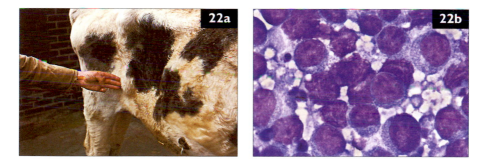

22 A Friesian cow (22a) presented because it was thin and was scouring. A hemispherical mass on its flank was aspirated and a smear made (22b) (Wright–Giemsa, ×100 oil).
a What cells are present?
b What is your diagnosis?

21 a Plasma cells represent the predominant cell population, characterized by a dense eccentric round nucleus and abundant blue cytoplasm. Many small to medium-sized lymphocytes and a few neutrophils (<2%) are present. Scattered large mononuclear phagocytes are easily noted. The cytoplasm of these cells contains 20–30 oval organisms approximately 3–5 μm in size with a red nucleus and pale blue cytoplasm representing amastigotes of *Leishmania infantum*. A red organelle, eccentric to the nucleus, is sometimes evident within the cytoplasm of these parasites. This is the kinetoplast, which is a distinctive feature of *Leishmania* organisms. This protozoal infection has a worldwide distribution and can cause different forms of disease in humans and animals (cutaneous, visceral and mucocutaneous). Different species are transmitted by various species of *Phlebotomus*, the sandfly.

Leishmania infantum is endemic in Mediterranean countries. Dogs are the main reservoir of the parasite. Infection in cats has been documented but is very rare. The promastigote is the parasitic stage in the sandfly, which infects the vertebrate host when bitten. Macrophages of the vertebrate host phagocytose the promastigotes, which starts intracellular replication as amastigotes. Macrophages die and release amastigotes, which enter other fixed or circulating macrophages. When a sandfly ingests blood containing infected macrophages from a vertebrate, amastigotes reproduce as promastigotes in the vector. Postinfection progression of the disease depends on host immune responses. Higher infectivity seems associated with lower proportions of T helper cells. Many studies confirm the high incidence of asymptomatic infections in dogs living in endemic areas.

Direct observation of the parasite in lymph nodes, bone marrow and skin aspirates/biopsy is the most reliable diagnostic test, but sensitivity is low (50–70%) and often no parasites can be detected. In these cases, cytology can be useful to exclude other diseases such as lymphoma, which have a similar clinical presentation.

b The endocellular parasite affects the mononuclear phagocyte system, often resulting in a strong immune system response and type III hypersensitivity (immune-complexes mediated), resulting in secondary renal, ocular, skin and synovial damage. Laboratory investigation often reveals marked hyperglobulinaemia and hypoalbuminaemia, renal insufficiency, nephrotic syndrome or glomerulonephritis. Serum protein electrophoresis is characterized by polyclonal gammopathy but monoclonal gammopathy has also been reported. Bleeding disorders are often observed in the course of canine leishmaniasis, particularly epistaxis. Epistaxis may be the only presenting sign, although thrombocytopenia is rarely observed. An acquired thrombocytopathy secondary to hyperglobulinaemia and hyperviscosity syndrome are hypothesized to be at the origin of this bleeding disorder.

22 a Apart from RBCs and occasional neutrophils, the smear contains an homogeneous population of pleomorphic round cells with thin margins of basophilic cytoplasm. Nuclei vary widely in size and they have irregular margins and clumped chromatin with prominent nucleoli.
b Lymphosarcoma.

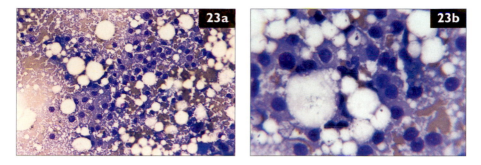

23 A 12-year-old neutered male DSH cat presented with polyuria and polydipsia, polyphagia, a pendulous abdomen, muscle wasting, alopecia, seborrhoea and urinary tract infection. ACTH stimulation and dexamethasone suppression testing confirmed hyperadrenocorticism. On ultrasonography, a right adrenal gland mass was identified. A unilateral adrenalectomy was performed and an impression smear of the mass prepared for cytological examination. The mass was submitted for histological evaluation.

a Describe the cytological features of the nucleated cells (23a, b) (Leishman's, ×40 and ×100 oil, respectively).

b What is the likely origin/type of these cells?

c Based on this group of cells, what diagnosis would you make in this case?

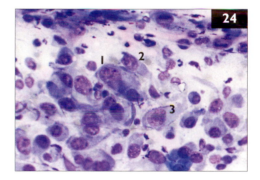

24 A six-year-old Golden Retriever has a rapidly growing, ill-defined mass above the left hock. The mass is subcutaneous and appears to extend circumferentially around the limb. The overlying skin is erythematous and beginning to ulcerate. An FNA is obtained (24) (Giemsa, ×100 oil).

a Describe and classify the cells illustrated.

b What criteria of malignancy are present?

c Can you suggest a likely diagnosis?

d What would you do next?

23 a There is a homogeneous population of mononuclear cells that have eccentric nuclei and abundant basophilic cytoplasm containing fine vacuoles. There are also some neutrophils and macrophages.

b The mononuclear cells are neuroendocrine in origin and do not demonstrate criteria of malignancy.

c The cytological diagnosis is adrenal hyperplasia/adrenal adenoma. The histopathological diagnosis was adrenocortical adenoma. In one report of 18 cases of hyperadrenocorticism, 14 cats were diagnosed with pituitary-dependent hyperadrenocorticism and four cats with a unilateral adrenocortical tumour (2 adrenocortical carcinomas, 2 adrenal adenomas).

Note: The identification of hyperadrenocorticism in this case was well supported by other laboratory data and the localization of a mass in the right adrenal gland was supportive of a tumour. In other cases the presence of an intra-abdominal mass may be the initial observation and ultrasound-guided fine needle aspiration may be the initial avenue of investigation. In those cases the organ or cell type of origin of the mass may not be clinically apparent. Some differences in the appearance of adrenal mass aspirates and impression smears should be kept in mind. In this case an impression smear shows primarily intact cells with the classic vacuolated appearance that is typical of adrenal gland origin. Aspirates from adrenal masses are reported to more commonly contain large numbers of nuclei that have been stripped of cytoplasm or which appear in a background of lightly basophilic cytoplasm with indistinct borders. This appearance is typical of neuroendocrine neoplasia. Intact cells similar to the ones illustrated in this case may also be present in variable numbers. If marked anaplasia or pleomorphic features consistent with malignancy are present, a diagnosis of a malignant neoplasia is possible. However, well-differentiated carcinomas may be difficult to distinguish from adenomas and additional histological evaluation and clinical investigation of possible metastasis may be needed to help distinguish adenomas from well-differentiated carcinomas.

24 a Some cells are discrete, while others are in small clusters with ill-defined margins. The cells vary in shape. Some are round; others are stellate (1). Some have blunt cytoplasmic tails extending away from the nucleus (2). The cells are mesenchymal cells.

b Numerous criteria of malignancy are present. There is marked anisocytosis and anisokaryosis. There is a variable, but often high, nuclear:cytoplasmic ratio. The nuclear chromatin is often stippled. There are several bi- and multinucleated cells. Some cells have multiple nucleoli in a large nucleus (3).

c The cells are mesenchymal and there are criteria of malignancy suggesting this is a sarcoma. The type of sarcoma cannot be reliably determined from cytology.

d This lesion looks aggressive clinically and cytologically and may require radical therapy. Therefore, a definitive diagnosis should be made before planning treatment and giving a prognosis. A biopsy should be taken for histological evaluation.

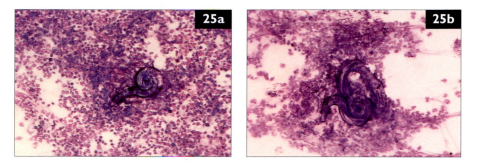

25 A two-year-old DSH cat presented with a history of coughing and gagging that appeared progressive and worsening in intensity. The cat was up-to-date on all vaccinations. A CBC with differential revealed a modest eosinophilia; there were no biochemical abnormalities. Thoracic radiographs revealed a diffuse interstitial pattern with focal peribronchial densities. A transtracheal wash was performed (25a, b) (Wright–Giemsa, ×10 and ×50 oil, respectively). What are the main differentials with this pulmonary pattern and peripheral eosinophilia?

26 A smear is made from an FNA collected from a submandibular lymph node of a 13-year-old female crossbred dog.

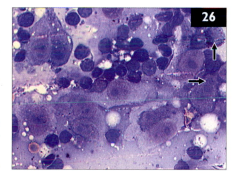

a Describe the cells seen in the smear (26) (Wright–Giemsa, ×50 oil). What is your interpretation?

b Using the cytological features of the metastatic cells, list the most likely differential diagnosis.

c Which special stains could you use to confirm your diagnosis?

d What are the sensitivity and specificity of fine needle aspiration of regional lymph nodes to determine possible metastasis, compared with histological examination of the entire node?

e Which tumours tend to metastasize to regional lymph nodes: carcinomas or sarcomas?

25 Differentials include migration of intestinal parasites, lungworm infection and allergic pneumonitis.

The lungworm in cats is *Aleurostronglylus abstrusus* and the intermediate hosts are snails and slugs. The disease process is often self-limiting, although some cats do require therapy. Literature reports on the use of ivermectin and fenbendazole are available. This cat was an indoor-outdoor cat that had been missing for one week, eight weeks prior to developing the cough. The prepatent period for *A. abstrusus* infection is 6–18 weeks.

26 a A population of large pleomorphic oval to spindle shaped cells have almost effaced the lymph node aspirate. They are generally scattered individually but in some areas there appears to be intercellular cohesion. Individual cells have a moderate nuclear:cytoplasmic ratio and generally contain a single oval nucleus (some bi- and trinucleated cells are also present). Nuclei vary from 4 to 16 RBCs in diameter and they have smooth chromatin and 1–2 giant nucleoli. They have moderate amounts of fine grey cytoplasm and a small percentage contain green/black round/rice-grain shaped granules (see arrows). Low numbers of small lymphocytes and mild evidence of haemodilution are present on a deeply basophilic background. These findings indicate a metastasis of a malignant neoplasm.
b Malignant melanoma (primary mucosal mass: confirmed as melanoma on histology section).
c Fontana–Masson Silver stain: can identify small amounts of melanin in largely amelanotic neoplasms; S100: has a poor sensitivity (i.e. if positive, then it is diagnostically useful; however, if negative, then a melanoma cannot be excluded); vimentin: immunoperoxidase stain that identifies a fibrillar protein in mesenchymal cells and melanocytes.
d Sensitivity 100%, specificity 96%; therefore, fine needle aspiration may be a reliable screening method for detection of lymph node metastasis in dogs and cats with solid tumours.
e Carcinomas tend to metastasize to lymph nodes; sarcomas typically metastasize via the haematogenous route rather than the lymphatic route.
Note: The sensitivity and specificity of lymph node aspiration in the identification of metastases of solid tumours in dogs and cats may vary, depending on a number of factors. Sampling of a lymph node should include multiple aspirations and redirections in order to increase the probability of obtaining malignant cells when only a small focus of metastasis is present. In addition, in some cases, tumours may 'skip' lymph nodes along the channels of normal drainage and may not be present in those lymph nodes closest to the tumour. Some cases will present with lymph node enlargement as the primary sign and the identification of nonlymphoid malignancy within the lymph node is the first indication of an occult tumour. Some lymph nodes in the region of tumours may be enlarged and appear reactive on cytological evaluation; the absence of malignant cells in these nodes cytologically or histologically does not rule out the possibility of more distant metastases.

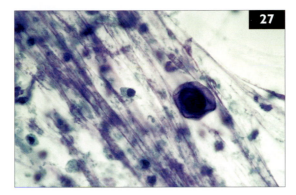

27 A ten-year-old Warmblood-cross gelding is referred for evaluation of worsening clinical signs associated with obstructive pulmonary disease/recurrent airway obstruction. A tracheal washing is collected by endoscope and smears prepared.
a What is the structure in the central right portion of this photomicrograph (27) (Papanicolaou, ×25)?
b What is its significance in a respiratory cytology specimen?

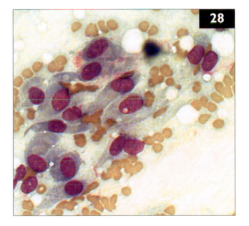

28 A seven-year-old neutered male Labrador Retriever presents with a slight limp. There is a multilobulated, apparently well-circumscribed, nonalopecic mass, measuring approximately 4 cm in diameter, involving the lateral aspect of the left hock area. Fine needle aspiration of the mass is performed and smears are prepared (28) (Wright's, ×100 oil).
a What is the most likely diagnosis?
b What therapeutic approach(es) can be recommended?

27 a A corpus amylacea. This is an acellular structure that could be confused with a cell since it has a densely staining centre that can be mistaken for a nucleus. The peripheral, concentric layers are less dense and should not be confused with cytoplasm. These bodies are thought to be composed of glycoproteins and they do not calcify. They are found in respiratory cytology specimens in humans with chronic alveolar oedema and/or obstruction due to cardiac insufficiency, pulmonary infarction and chronic bronchitis. They may be seen in low numbers in respiratory specimens from horses, dogs and cats with similar conditions.
b The corpus amylacea is significant since it supports the history of chronic obstruction. Casts of inspissated mucus with many embedded neutrophils were seen in other fields of this tracheal washing smear and provided additional cytological support for mechanical obstruction of airways.

28 a The cytological characteristics and location of the mass are compatible with haemangiopericytoma, a common skin tumour in dogs. The spindle cells tend to be plump, occurring singly or in bundles, with ovoid, single and occasionally multiple nuclei (not illustrated). The cells tend to possess feathered 'tails' and the cytoplasm is usually lightly to moderately basophilic and may contain a few discrete vacuoles. Generally, mild to moderate anisocytosis and anisokaryosis are present. The origin of these tumours is uncertain. They appear to be associated with the periphery of blood vessels (pericytes) and may be related to peripheral nerve sheath tumours. These tumours tend to be solitary and locally invasive, although they may appear well-circumscribed. Although metastasis is uncommon, recurrence following surgery is common, especially if the excision is incomplete.
b Because of the need for wide margins during excision, surgery may need to be repeated. Wide margins may be difficult to obtain because of the location of the mass (limb, often in the vicinity of a joint). This results in a high incidence of recurrence (up to 60% of cases); therefore, amputation or radiation therapy may be considered as alternative or complementary therapies, respectively.
Note: This case is illustrative of a spindle cell tumour that does not have extremely aggressive morphological features. The degree of atypia may vary in tumours of this type, depending on the rate of growth, whether they are ulcerated and whether or not there has been previous removal. Often a diagnosis of spindle cell tumour is as specific a diagnosis as can be made; in some cases there may be a high index of suspicion of haemangiopericytoma or schwannoma based on the location and features of the cells, and this diagnosis can be suggested with a high degree of confidence. Differential diagnoses include cutaneous fibrosarcoma or other types of sarcoma. The biological behaviour (high rate of local recurrence with low or infrequent metastasis) is similar in many types of cutaneous spindle cell tumours, so cytological identification is important and wide and deep surgical excision is indicated to help increase the probability of complete removal. In many cases, histological evaluation is needed to confirm the tumour type.

29 A six-year-old female spayed DSH cat presented for chronic weight loss and a recent history of vomiting and severe lethargy. Physical examination revealed pale, icteric mucous membranes. The temperature was 38°C (100.4°F) and pulse and respiration rates were slightly increased. Abdominal palpation and radiographs revealed diffuse hepatomegaly. Examin-

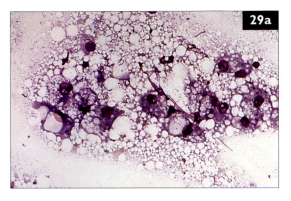

ation of a peripheral blood smear indicated RBC shape abnormalities including severe acanthocytosis. Abnormal biochemistry values were: AST = 150 U/l (ref. = 2–36 U/l); ALT = 350 U/l (ref. = 6–80 U/l); ALP = 135 U/l (ref. = 2–43 U/l); bilirubin = 68 µmol/l (ref. = 0–3.4 µmol/l). An FNA of the liver was obtained and a smear made (29a) (Wright–Giemsa, ×25).
a Explain the abnormal RBC shape and the biochemistry abnormalities.
b Describe the cytological findings, and give your cytological interpretation.
c List the differentials for your diagnosis, and discuss treatment options.

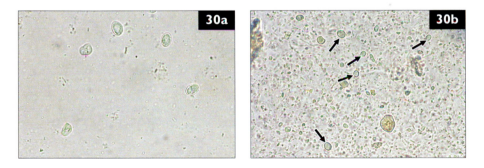

30 A 16-week-old Shih Tzu presented with mucoid diarrhoea. The puppy was outwardly well and had a good appetite. A zinc sulphate faecal float (×40) was made (30a). A saline mount (×40) was made for comparison (30b).
a What are these organisms?
b Describe how and where to look on the zinc sulphate faecal float to find the cysts.
c Are yeast cells larger or smaller than these cysts? Do they float?

29 a Acanthocytes are spherical erythrocytes with blunt tipped spicules of different lengths projecting from the surface at irregular intervals. Abnormal amounts of lipid may accumulate in the outer half of the lipid bilayer during liver disease. This causes the membrane to evaginate and form spicules, resulting in acanthocytosis. The mild elevation in ALT and AST suggests minimal hepatic damage. Elevated bilirubin and alkaline

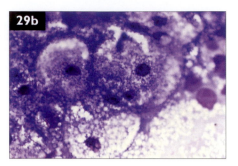

phosphatase are indicative of cholestatic liver disease. Even mild elevations of serum ALP are significant in the cat because of the short half-life of the enzyme in this species.

b Several hepatocytes are seen, many of which contain distinct, punctate, clear cytoplasmic vacuoles. The nuclei of many of these hepatocytes are pushed to the periphery due to cytoplasmic vacuoles. Abundant punctate vacuoles are also noted in the background. The cytological interpretation is vacuolar degeneration compatible with hepatic lipidosis.

c Hepatic lipidosis in cats may be a primary disease or may occur secondary to other metabolic, inflammatory or neoplastic conditions. Approximately 50% of cases are idiopathic. Differentials for secondary hepatic lipidosis include diabetes mellitus, pancreatitis, hyperthyroidism, steroids or neoplasia. The key to successful management of cats with lipidosis, as seen in this case, is early diagnosis and intensive nutritional support. Cats typically require nutritional support for 3–6 weeks with high-protein, calorie-dense food, usually via PEG tubes. Because these cats are already ill and stressed, extreme care must be taken not to cause further stress by force-feeding.

Note: An additional photomicrograph is included here for comparison (29b) (Wright–Giemsa, ×100 oil). The multiple small, crisply defined cytoplasmic vacuoles within hepatocytes are characteristic of this condition.

30 a *Giardia* species cysts.

b First check the entire slide for other parasite ova routinely at ×100. This gives the *Giardia* cysts time to float to the top of the zinc sulphate solution. Increase magnification and scan carefully, just under the cover slip – air bubbles, especially small ones, are a useful landmark for finding the very top of the solution droplet beneath a cover slip. *Giardia* cysts, when they are numerous, will all be in the same plane of focus.

c Yeast cells are very commonly mistaken for *Giardia* cysts, but are slightly smaller. Yeast will tend to sink to the bottom of the droplet.

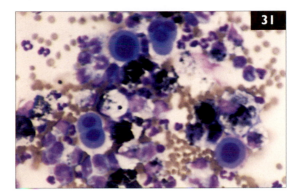

31 An 11-year-old mongrel dog has been losing weight and is dyspnoeic. Serosanguineous fluid is withdrawn from the pleural space (TP = 34 g/l, NCC = 10.6×10^9/l). A cytospun smear is made from the fluid (31) (Wright–Giemsa, ×50 oil).
a What cells are present?
b What is the fluid classification?
c What is your diagnosis?

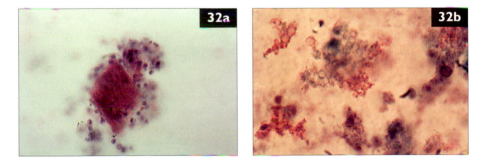

32 A seven-year-old horse used for three-day eventing is evaluated on the treadmill with endoscopy in place. Fresh blood is observed in the tracheal mucus as the horse is exercised. Exercise is discontinued. A tracheal washing is collected the following day and smears prepared.
a What is illustrated in the smears (32a, b) (Papanicolaou, ×20 and ×100 oil, respectively)?
b What is the significance of these findings?

	Transudate	Modified transudate	Exudate
Total protein (g/l)	<25	>25	>30
NCC ($\times 10^9$/l)	<1.5	<5	>5
Predominant cell type	Mesothelial cells Macrophages	Mesothelial cells Macrophages	Neutrophils Macrophages

31 a A mixed cell population is present, consisting of RBCs, neutrophils, macrophages and reactive mesothelial cells. A lot of black pigment is present extracellularly and intracellularly within the macrophages. This is melanin and the macrophages are melanophages.
b An exudate. (Guidelines for fluid classification in dogs and cats are shown above.)
c Metastatic melanoma.

32 a There is a cast of mucoproteinaceous material containing many erythrocytes in **32a**. The erythrocytes stain red-orange. Note the smooth sides of the cast indicative of formation within an airway. The ends (upper left and lower right) are jagged. Such a cast is consistent with recent haemorrhage. Based on studies of horses with blood instilled into the lung and those with respiratory cytology collected at known intervals following pulmonary haemorrhage, this appearance can be found 1–3 days following blood instillation or pulmonary haemorrhage. Finding of erythrocytes in a cast is unusual; more often, erythrocytes are seen as discrete cells in the background of the smear.

There are lysed, crenated and fragmented erythrocytes, often in clumps, in **32b**. This is typical of erythrocytes associated with blood instillation or pulmonary haemorrhage that has occurred 1–3 days previously. Sometimes, blood contamination will include lysed and intact erythrocytes, but the clumped, crenated and fragmented appearance is typical of 'ageing' blood and should raise the suspicion of recent pathological haemorrhage.

b The significance of these findings relates to recent pulmonary haemorrhage, probably within the last 1–3 days. The cast of material or presence of lysed, crenated and fragmented erythrocytes in clumps is supportive of pathological haemorrhage rather than contamination with blood at collection. The finding of a few, single fresh erythrocytes may be within normal limits in a respiratory cytology specimen. Contamination with blood due to mild trauma during collection usually results in single, discrete erythrocytes that are lysed or intact. Contamination with blood is an unusual finding in cases with routine collections. It is more common if the animal is fractious or if there is difficulty that results in endoscopic trauma to the airways. Communication with the cytologist regarding difficult collections or those with a high probability of traumatic contamination is recommended.

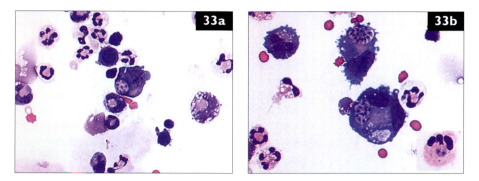

33 A cat presented with pyrexia, pneumonia and dyspnoea. Pleural fluid was obtained and smears made from sediment from the fluid. Similar findings were also obtained from bronchoalveolar lavage.

a Identify the aetiological agent in this exudative effusion, with precise reference to the exact stage of its life cycle as seen in these photomicrographs (33a, b) (Wright–Giemsa, ×50 and ×100 oil, respectively).

b What other laboratory tests would you like to use to support your cytological suspicion?

c Given the following laboratory results, what can you determine about the kinetics of *Toxoplasma gondii* from these values: IgM – ELISA ~ 1:256; IgG – ELISA ~ 1:64?

d Toxoplasmosis is a potential zoonotic risk. Are cat owners and veterinarians at significantly higher risk than the general population of acquiring *T. gondii* infection?

e Are seropositive cats a risk for pregnant women or immunocompromised individuals?

34 A ten-year-old entire male Beagle presents with multiple nodular enlargements surrounding the anus. This is associated with ulceration and bleeding and is accompanied by a disagreeable odour. Fine needle aspiration is performed and smears prepared (34) (Wright's, ×100 oil).

a What is the most likely diagnosis?

b What therapy would you recommend?

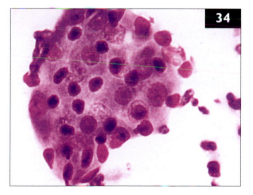

33 a Intracellular protozoon consistent with *Toxoplasma gondii*. Stage: tachyzoites, multiplying within macrophages and neutrophils (insert lower right corner, **33b**).
b Serology.
c IgM antibodies can identify early infection at 1–2 weeks post exposure. They peak at 3–6 weeks and usually drop to negative at 12 weeks post exposure. Caution: some cats can have sporadic low IgM ELISA titres for up to one year post exposure. IgG antibodies develop at approximately two weeks post infection and can remain high for several years to the life of the cat. Based on the high IgM titre and presence of IgG, this patient has an active, progressing to established *T. gondii* infection. A diagnosis of active infection can also be made by a four-fold increase in serial IgG tests 2–3 weeks apart.
d No. Minimizing risk does not have to include prevention of exposure to cats but must prevent exposure to oocysts (particularly sporulated oocysts). Therefore, pregnant women and immunocompromised individuals should not change cat litter boxes, should wear gloves when gardening and should maintain extra hygiene when working with food products, particularly raw meat. Only sporulated oocysts are infective; therefore, litter must be changed daily and, given cats' fastidious grooming habits, they are unlikely to be a risk since they do not have sporulated oocysts on their fur.
e No. Most seropositive cats have completed the oocyst shedding period and are unlikely to repeat shedding (for up to six years).

34 a The clinical signs, signalment and cytological observations are most consistent with perianal adenoma. This tumour is most common in older, sexually intact dogs (>8 years of age). Multiple tumours in the area around the anus are common, as are bleeding and ulcerative lesions. These tumours are rarely malignant in males.
b Surgical excision is recommended. Castration will arrest tumour growth and should be done at the same time, as this tumour is testosterone dependent. Oestrogen therapy is recommended in cases in which the tumour cannot be completely removed, and it may also be used following surgery as adjunct therapy. Antibiotic therapy may be needed if concomitant infection is suspected.
Note: The cytological features of perianal adenoma are classic in this case. The cells are typically large and resemble hepatocytes and are referred to as 'hepatoid'. They typically have round, central nuclei with single, distinct nucleoli and moderate to abundant, oval to angular cytoplasm. They usually occur in cohesive groups. In some cases, small 'reserve' cells also may be apparent mixed with the larger hepatoid cells. There may be concurrent inflammation and/or haemorrhage. Perianal adenocarcinoma is less common and exhibits more bizarre and/or variable features compatible with malignancy. It may present as a relatively undifferentiated malignancy cytologically and require surgical biopsy and histological evaluation to confirm cell type of origin.

35 A 12-year-old mare is referred because of a history of chronic infertility over a two-year period. She has a history of having a foal each year since she was six years old, but has failed to produce a foal following breeding for the last two years. The mare has been cultured and treated for bacterial infection with infusion of antibiotics on multiple cycles prior to referral. A uterine washing is collected as part of the reproductive work up.

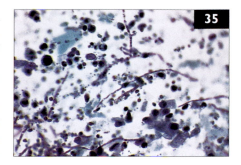

a What cellular and noncellular features are apparent in this smear of sediment from the uterine washing (35) (Papanicolaou, ×20)?
b What is your interpretation of the smear?

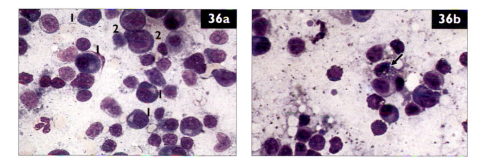

36 An eight-year-old crossbred dog has a history of crusting, flaky skin lesions, weight loss, lethargy and polyarthropathy. There is generalized, moderate lymphadenopathy. The dog was imported from Spain 18 months previously. Smears from FNAs from two lymph nodes are shown (36a, b) (both Giemsa, ×100 oil).
a What cell(s) are increased in number in 36a?
b What does this indicate?
c What is the cell next to the arrowhead in 36b?
d Given the history and clinical signs, can you speculate on a possible cause for the generalized lymphadenopathy?

35 a There are some clumps of blue-green mucus with necrotic debris and scattered columnar epithelial cells. The linear structures are fragments of fungal hyphae.
b The interpretation is cytological grade IV associated with severe inflammation and necrosis associated with uterine fungal infection. This grade represents a marked deviation from normal. Uterine cytology grades have some prognostic significance, since mares with grade IV cytology have a decreased pregnancy rate following treatment compared with mares with lower grades. Grade I cytology is within normal limits, grade II is a slight deviation from normal and grade III is a moderate deviation from normal.

The repeated antibiotic treatment likely predisposed this mare to development of fungal infection. *Candida albicans* is the most commonly reported cause of equine fungal endometritis, but a variety of opportunistic fungi may be implicated in uterine infections.

36 a Plasma cells (1). These cells have eccentric nuclei and a perinuclear clear area, which is the Golgi area, the site of immunoglobulin production. There also appear to be increased numbers of lymphoblasts (2).
b This indicates reactive hyperplasia and particularly plasma cell hyperplasia.
c A 'Mott cell'. This is a plasma cell containing Russell bodies, which are accumulations of immunoglobulins within vesicles.
d Plasma cell hyperplasia is caused by chronic antigenic stimulation. In this case the cause was *Leishmania* infection. The organisms were identified in macrophages in a bone marrow aspirate.
Note: Other cases in this book illustrate *Leishmania* organisms and lymphoid and plasma cell hyperplasia and Mott cells. This case is included to emphasize recognition of basic processes and underlying mechanisms contributing to this cytological appearance. Knowledge of the significance of the finding of hyperplasia, with the history of importation from Spain, indicated that additional investigation was required to identify the suspected organism. Other differential diagnoses for chronic immune stimulation that could result in this appearance cytologically include chronic parasitic, fungal, bacterial or protozoal infections. Tick-borne diseases should be included in the differential in those countries or areas where tick exposure may be present. Sometimes, chronic, noninfectious diseases processes, including neoplasia, systemic lupus erythematosus or immune-mediated disease involving the skin and/or joints, could present with this appearance. Therefore, an extensive work up may be required in some cases in order to determine the most likely underlying cause. The cytological evaluation is part of this work up.

37 A weanling foal presented with pyrexia, moderate mucopurulent nasal discharge and wheezes and crackles on thoracic auscultation. A tracheal washing was collected.
a What are the cells shown in this photomicrograph (37a) (Sano's modification of Pollack's Trichrome, ×50 oil)?
b What is the significance of this finding?

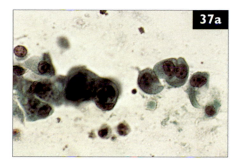

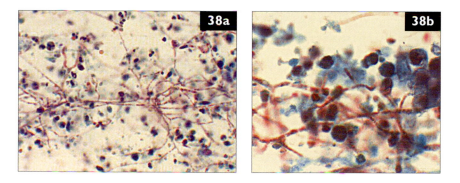

38 An eight-year-old broodmare (three previous foals) presents with a history of repeated uterine infections that had been treated with antibiotics. A uterine washing is collected to determine the mare's status.
a Describe the features shown (38a, b) (Papanicolaou, ×50 oil and ×100 oil, respectively).
b What is your interpretation of these findings?
c What is the significance of these findings?

39 A six-year-old neutered male mixed breed dog presented for routine vaccinations. A faecal flotation sample had many of these large, symmetrical sausage-shaped organisms (39) (unstained zinc sulphate flotation sample, ×40).
a Is this a parasite?
b What is it?

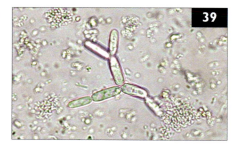

45

37 **a** Moderately to markedly atypical columnar epithelial cells. Their nuclei are enlarged and have increased chromatin prominence. Small but distinct nucleoli are visible in several of the cells. Intercellular cohesion is observable, but cilia are not seen and normal orderly orientation and polarity of the cells are not preserved. Compare the features with those in 37b (equine tracheal washing, Sano's

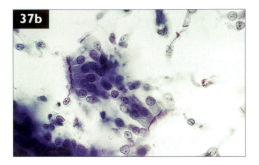

modification of Pollack's Trichrome, ×50 oil). In this photomicrograph there is a cohesive group of columnar epithelial cells whose features are within normal limits. The nuclei are basal and uniform with delicate chromatin. Nucleoli are absent or inconspicuous. The terminal bar with attached cilia is easily seen at the luminal aspect of the columnar epithelial cells.

b The epithelial atypia is significant since it indicates chronic, severe irritation to the airways. Without normal cells and cilia, the mucociliary apparatus and clearance mechanisms of the lung are compromised. In other fields there were numerous neutrophils. The features supported the clinical diagnosis of severe, chronic bronchopneumonia.

38 **a** There are a few columnar epithelial cells with a mat of intertwining fungal hyphae. The hyphae are narrow and septate.
b These findings are consistent with a fungal infection of the equine uterus.
c The diagnosis indicates that specific antifungal treatment is needed.

   Candida species are frequently the cause of uterine fungal infections but a number of opportunistic fungi may be involved in uterine infections.

39 **a** No, it is a fairly common pseudoparasite in dog faeces.
b A yeast, *Saccharomycopsis gutulatus*. Owners report that many dogs that pass this organism eat rabbit faeces.

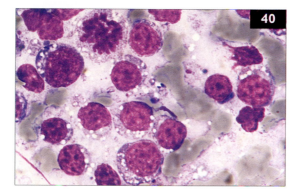

40 An FNA is collected from a canine lymph node.
a Describe the cells represented in this photomicrograph (40) (May–Grünwald–Giemsa, ×100 oil).
b What is your diagnosis, and what are the differential diagnoses?

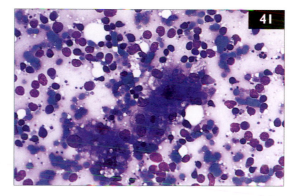

41 An eight-year-old female spayed DSH cat presented with a two-week history of intermittent vomiting. There was an acute onset of lethargy and anorexia. Significant findings on physical examination included icterus and severe hepatomegaly. CBC findings included moderate, nonregenerative anaemia (PCV = 0.23 l/l). Abnormal biochemistry findings were: ALT = 360 U/l (ref. = 10–80 U/l); ALP = 120 U/L (ref. = 2–43 U/l); bilirubin = 55 μmol/l (ref. = 0–3.4 μmol/l). An FNA of the liver was obtained and a smear made (41) (Wright–Giemsa, ×25).
a Describe the cytological findings, and give your cytological interpretation.
b Discuss the condition.
c Discuss the prognosis and treatment options.

40 a An atypical proliferation of lymphoid cells that are relatively uniform in size and shape (small/medium sized). In some cells the nucleus exhibits irregularly clumped chromatin associated with clearly visible nucleoli. The cytoplasm is moderate, well-defined and deeply basophilic and contains abundant clear vacuoles. A mitosis at the top suggests a high mitotic index.
b Diagnosis: small-cell high-grade lymphoma (Burkitt-like type) (B-cell phenotype: CD79a+, CD3-). Differential diagnoses: none with benign hyperplasia; centroblastic polymorphic (CBP) lymphoma, but the relatively uniform size, clumped chromatin and vacuoles are unusual for CBP lymphomas.

41 a The smear contains several hepatocytes with round to oval nuclei and light basophilic cytoplasm. A single distinct prominent nucleolus characteristic of hepatocytes is also present. Large numbers of well-differentiated lymphocytes are present around the hepatocytes and in the background. Lymphocytes are discrete cells with a small amount of cytoplasm. Nuclei are round and are about one to one and a half times the size of erythrocytes. Nuclear chromatin is dense and clumped. The cytological interpretation is a well-differentiated hepatic lymphoma.
b Many cats with hepatic lymphoma will present cytologically with an abundant population of small, well-differentiated lymphocytes. It is important to differentiate lymphocytic periportal hepatitis from hepatic lymphoma. Cats with hepatic lymphoma usually have severe hepatomegaly, whereas with lymphocytic periportal hepatitis, hepatomegaly is typically mild. Histological confirmation is recommended in cats with severe lymphocytic infiltrates and marked hepatomegaly, regardless of the cytological appearance of the lymphocytes.
c Treatment options include chemotherapy. In a few isolated cases where the tumour is localized and easily accessible, surgery or radiation therapy may be used. A combination of chemotherapeutic drugs, including doxorubicin, cyclophosphamide and vincristine, and prednisone, administered over many weeks is the most common course of treatment. During the course of treatment leukocyte and erythrocyte numbers are closely monitored. The remission and survival rates of cats with lymphoma vary depending on the cat's FeLV status, the location of the tumour(s) and how quickly the tumour is diagnosed and treated. In general, about 70% of cats will respond to the chemotherapy protocol. On average, these cats will live an additional 4–6 months. However, about 30–40% of the cats that respond will go into a more complete remission that can last for two years or longer. Cats that are not treated have an average survival time of only 4–6 weeks once the diagnosis has been made.
Note: As pointed out above, the small lymphocytes illustrated in this case do not have features associated with classical lymphoid malignancy (large numbers of large lymphocytes and lymphoblasts) as is usually seen in the dog. It is important to include well-differentiated or so-called 'small cell' lymphoma in your differential diagnosis list in addition to lymphocytic periportal hepatitis when lymphocytes are numerous in a hepatic aspirate.

42 A 16-week-old entire male Golden Retriever presented with a one-day history of vomiting, diarrhoea, anorexia, lethargy and fever (40°C [104°F]). The puppy had been given three distemper/adenovirus/paramyxovirus/parvovirus vaccines but had not yet been vaccinated against rabies. A parvovirus ELISA was negative. A direct faecal smear was made (**42**) (Gram's, ×100 oil).

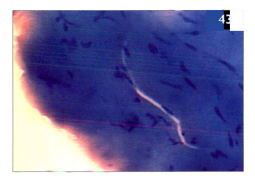

a Describe the organisms indicated by the arrows.
b What might these organisms be?
c What other tests are likely to aid your diagnosis?

43 An FNA is collected from a firm mass on the neck of a seven-year-old Welsh cob gelding.

a Describe the structure shown in the smear (**43**) (Wright–Giemsa, ×100 oil).
b What is your interpretation?
c What are your differential diagnoses?

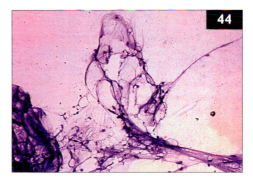

44 A 13-year old spayed female Miniature Poodle presents with two mobile, soft, well-circumscribed, subcutaneous sternal masses, 3 cm and 6 cm in diameter, respectively. The owner had noticed one mass three months previously. Fine needle aspiration of both masses is performed and smears are prepared. A representative field of both specimens is illustrated (**44**) (Wright's, ×20). What is your diagnosis?

42 a They are tiny, curved gram-negative (pink) rods, in short chains of two and three.

b *Campylobacter* species look like this on a faecal Gram's stain. They are much more difficult to visualize than many appreciate. The term 'seagulls' has been used to describe the short chains of 'C'-shaped bacteria that resemble (but are not) spirochaetes.

c Faecal culture is the gold standard to demonstrate *Campylobacter* (though it can also be cultured from some asymptomatic dogs' faeces). When present in large numbers, a saline wet-mount of faeces observed at ×40 shows the 'swarm-of-bees' motility characteristic of these tiny organisms.

Note: Special media may be supplied by the laboratory for culture of *Campylobacter* species. It is important to check with the laboratory regarding media and sample requirements prior to submission.

43 a There is a large blue-staining structure containing multiple, oval, elongated nuclei. Nucleoli are not recognized. In some areas, multiple parallel striations or 'stripes' are seen perpendicular to the long axis of the structure.

b This structure is a striated (skeletal) muscle fragment.

c If present in small numbers, the possibility of spurious aspiration of muscle should be considered. If present in large numbers, the possibility of a rhabdomyoma should be considered.

44 The cells depicted are well-differentiated adipocytes. These cells are large, appear in aggregates or sometimes singly, and contain fat that stains negatively with Wright's, such that the cytoplasm appears clear. The cells possess a small, round or ovoid, pyknotic nucleus that may be compressed and located in the periphery of the cell. This benign tumour is a lipoma, which is common in dogs. If the mass hinders the animal, or the owner, it may be removed surgically. Infiltrative lipomas, and their malignant counterpart, liposarcomas, are less common. When sampling for cytology, frequently the first indication that a lipoma has been aspirated is the clear, oily appearance of the material ejected from the aspiration needle onto the slide. Care must be taken while staining to ensure that the material does not wash off the slide, as fat does not adhere readily to the glass surface.

Note: Gentle heat fixing of greasy material to a slide may be of benefit in keeping adipose cells adherent to slides during staining. This can be accomplished by holding a slide over a Bunsen burner or lighter or gentle heating on a heating tray/bar for a few seconds so that the side opposite to that containing the cellular material is slowly warmed. The slide must be left to cool completely before staining. Slides coated with poly-l-lysine, which are used for Papanicolaou staining and/or increased adherence of tissue sections to slides, are also helpful in promoting cellular adherence and eliminating loss of cells during staining.

Sometimes, local fat will be aspirated and cannot be reliably differentiated from the adipose cells of a lipoma. If there is any doubt as to the presence of a discrete mass, surgical removal with histological evaluation is recommended.

45 A pleural fluid specimen is submitted from a three-year-old neutered female Siamese cat that presented with dyspnoea of recent onset and pleural effusion.
a Describe the features shown in the smear (45) (Wright–Giemsa, ×50 oil).
b What is your interpretation of these findings?
c What differential diagnoses should you consider?

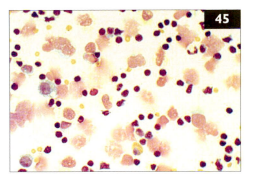

46 The owner of a five-year-old neutered male Boxer has noticed a subcutaneous mass in the cervical region of his pet. No other lesions are apparent. The mass is located on the dorsal aspect of the neck, behind the left ear. It measures approximately 5 cm in diameter and is poorly circumscribed, adherent and firm. The regional lymph nodes are not enlarged. Fine needle aspiration is performed and smears are prepared (46) (Wright's, ×100 oil).
a What is the most likely diagnosis?
b What further diagnostic work up do you recommend?
c What therapy do you recommend?

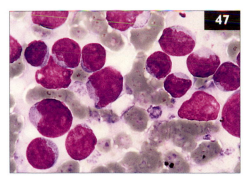

47 An FNA is collected from a canine lymph node.
a Describe the cells represented in this photomicrograph (47) (May–Grünwald–Giemsa, ×100 oil).
b What is your diagnosis, and what are the differential diagnoses?

51

45 a There are a few erythrocytes and a moderate number of smudged and ruptured cells that cannot be identified. There are a moderate number of intact cells. The majority of these are small, mature lymphocytes. A few neutrophils, eosinophils and macrophages are seen.
b This is a lymphocytic effusion. This appearance is often seen with chylous effusions. Chylous effusions can appear slightly haemolysed and 'milky' macroscopically.
c The predominance of small lymphocytes is suggestive of lymph stasis. Differentials should include the possibility of cardiac insufficiency or an intrathoracic mass (abscess, haematoma, granuloma or tumour) that is interfering with venous/lymphatic return but not shedding diagnostic elements into the pleural fluid. Ruptured thoracic duct, diaphragmatic hernia with organ displacement and idiopathic effusions may also have this appearance but are less common.

46 a The cytological findings are consistent with a mast cell tumour. Although not observed in this case, eosinophils may be present with mast cell neoplasia.
b Histological examination is necessary to grade the tumour. Some tumours that appear well-differentiated and thus benign on cytological examination may exhibit malignant morphology in histological sections.
c If grading shows the tumour to be benign, surgical treatment is usually sufficient. Careful examination of lymph nodes should be performed in order to rule out metastasis, even if no other lesions are apparent. A complete work up includes: complete blood count, clinical chemistry panel, urinalysis, lymph node cytology and radiographs or ultrasound to check for metastases.
Note: Previous recommendations to include buffy coat smears for examination for metastatic mast cell tumours have proved to be unreliable. There are some cases of mast cell tumour in which granules stain poorly or not at all with Diff-Quik. This should be borne in mind when mast cell tumour is suspected but the cytological appearance is that of a 'round cell tumour' and metachromatic granules are absent or sparse. Evaluation of smears stained with Wright–Giemsa or Romanowsky stains other than Diff-Quik is indicated to determine if there may be more prominent granule staining.

Mast cell tumours from cats may exhibit more marked variation in cellular morphology and degree of granulation and granule staining than that usually seen in dogs. The behaviour of cutaneous mast cell tumours in cats is usually benign and is not associated with the potential for aggressive biological behaviour that is more commonly seen in canine mast cell tumours.

47 a A mixture of small, medium-sized and large lymphoid cells. The nuclei have very irregular outlines, fine chromatin and non-prominent clear nucleoli, more visible in the largest cells. The cytoplasm is moderately extended and pale or poorly basophilic.
b Diagnosis: pleomorphic mixed lymphoma (T-cell phenotype: CD3+, CD4+, CD79a–). Differential diagnoses: atypical T-cell hyperplasia – the lack of mixing with normal lymphocytes is in favour of a lymphoma; none with another type of lymphoma.

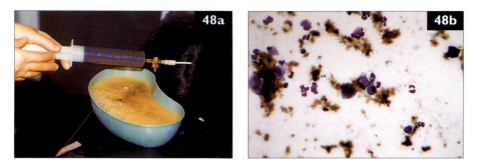

48 A two-year-old Labrador Retriever was involved in a road traffic accident. He sustained no fractures and was treated only for shock. Over the following three weeks there was a slow but progressive increase in abdominal size and the dog became depressed. Abdominocentesis produced approximately five litres of dark green/brown fluid (48a). The fluid was submitted to a diagnostic laboratory where direct smears were made for cytological examination (48b) (Wright–Giemsa, ×100 oil).
a Describe the background of the smear.
b Identify the cells present.
c What is your provisional diagnosis, and what other tests may be used to confirm this diagnosis?

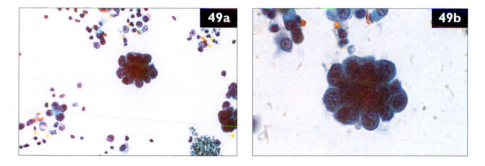

49 An eight-year-old female Siamese cat presented with periodic dyspnoea and sneezing.
a Describe the features shown in these smears (49a, b) (Papanicolaou, ×50 oil and ×100 oil, respectively).
b What is the significance of the cluster of cells in the upper central portion of each of these figures?
c Comment on the features seen. What other possible differentials should be considered?

48 a There is a large amount of golden-brown granular material present. This is bile pigment, which may be intracellular or extracellular. It can vary in colour from golden-brown to blue-green.

b There is a mixed population of macrophages and degenerate neutrophils. However, in this case the delay in preparation of smears of the fluid may have contributed to the loss of neutrophil nuclear integrity.

c The gross appearance of the fluid and the cytological features are typical of a biliary peritonitis. The cellular response in such cases is very variable, but the presence of bile usually results in an inflammatory response. Comparison of the bilirubin concentration in the serum and fluid may aid in the diagnosis. The fluid may be sterile or septic. No bacteria were isolated in this case and the trauma to the common bile duct was repaired surgically. The patient made an uneventful recovery.

Note: Bile pigment may range from golden-brown to yellow or blue-green in Wright–Giemsa and Papanicolaou-stained smears of bilious effusions. In some smears it may have a granular purple appearance and it may be difficult to distinguish unless there is some green to golden-brown material that suggests bile pigment. It may vary in amount, depending on the degree of damage, amount of bile leakage and duration of the condition. Because it is noncellular, bile pigment may be easily overlooked if not present in large amounts, or confused with other sources of pigment or precipitate, such as haemorrhage. Correct identification and recognition of its significance provide valuable information that can initiate additional confirmatory testing and and thus provide a timely assessment before attempts to repair the underlying damage to the biliary system.

49 a There are a few erythrocytes, neutrophils and macrophages. In the lower left corner of **49a** there is a large macrophage that contains phagocytosed mucus. There are scattered columnar to low columnar epithelial cells. In the upper central portion of the figures there is a cluster of cohesive cells consistent with epithelial origin. These cells have oval, basal or eccentric nuclei, often with increased chromatin prominence. The cytoplasm is moderate and stains darkly. A few neutrophils are present.

b The cluster of cells is consistent with a reactive proliferation of small airway epithelium. It is significant as a reflection of bronchiolitis.

c The cytological features are not specific but are consistent with an active (neutrophilic) inflammatory condition with irritation to small airways (bronchiolitis). These are nonspecific findings but they may occur with a variety of conditions. Differentials should include infectious or noninfectious conditions that may cause chronic irritation and inflammation.

50 A seven-year-old half-bred mare was unthrifty and eating poorly. A sample of peritoneal fluid was yellow, mildly turbid and had an NCC of 27 ×10⁹/l and a TP of 47 g/l. A cytospun smear of the fluid was made (50a) (Wright–Giemsa, ×100 oil). On rectal examination a spherical mass was palpated in mid-abdomen. Fluid from the mass was aspirated under ultrasound guidance and a smear was made from the fluid (50b) (Wright–Giemsa, ×100 oil).

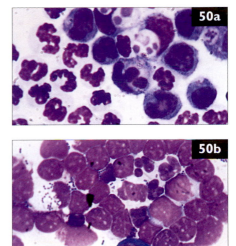

a What type of fluid (fluid classification) is present in the abdomen?
b What are the cells shown in 50a?
c What are the cells shown in 50b?
d What is your diagnosis?

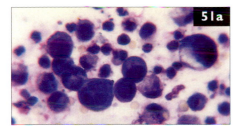

51 A 14-year-old male DSH cat presented with a three-month history of weight loss and dyspnoea. Physical examination and diagnostic imaging identified a pleural effusion and the presence of a right middle lung lobe mass. Thoracocentesis was performed and 50 ml of yellow, slightly turbid fluid was obtained (TP = 40 g/l; NCC = 3.4 × 10⁹/l). Cytospin prepara-

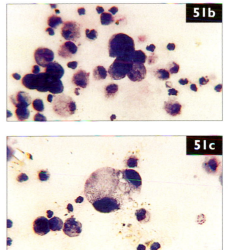

tions were made from the pleural fluid specimen (51a, b, c) (Leishman's, all ×100 oil).
a Based on the fluid analysis results, how would you classify this fluid?
b Based on the groups of cells, what diagnosis would you make in this case?

50 a An exudate.
b Neutrophils and reactive macrophages and lymphocytes. The macrophages contain ingested nuclear material. Microorganisms are not seen.
c The cell at the bottom centre is a lymphoblast and many of the remainder have the appearance of round cells, with cellular moulding. However, three cells in the centre are neutrophils and many of the others are considered to be karyolysed neutrophils. Numerous coccoid microorganisms are also present.
d Subacute/chronic peritonitis. This animal was found to have an encapsulated intra-abdominal abscess.
Note: Reference values for NCCs and classification of effusions in large animals differ from those for small animal specimens. (Guidelines for fluid classification in cows and horses are shown in question **3**.)

This case illustrates the importance of considering the proportions and absolute numbers of cell types and all the features in cytological preparations. The finding of a few lymphoblasts and some features suggestive of malignancy does not confirm the presence of malignancy, although it may raise the possibility of neoplasia.

The finding of many karyolytic neutrophils and intracellular bacterial cocci is consistent with an infectious and inflammatory condition. Intra-abdominal abscess should be considered when peritonitis is present. In some cases the abscess may be encapsulated and cause changes associated with irritation, while in others it may rupture or leak into the peritoneal cavity (as this case likely did) or contribute to generalized sepsis.

51 a A modified transudate (see Table in answer **31**).
b Some neutrophils and macrophages are present. There is a distinct population of larger cells that appear individually and in small clumps and show anisocytosis, hyperchromic nuclei, multinucleation, prominent nucleoli, abnormal mitosis and basophilic macrovacuolated cytoplasm. These cells are epithelial in origin and show characteristics of malignancy (carcinoma cells). An exploratory thoracotomy was performed and the right middle lung lobe was removed. The histopathological diagnosis was pulmonary adenocarcinoma.
Note: The cytological diagnosis of adenocarcinoma metastatic to pleural fluid is not specific as to the primary site of origin. In this case, pulmonary adenocarcinoma was the primary site. The malignant cells illustrated in these figures show rounding up typical of cells that have exfoliated into a body cavity effusion. The range of features and degree of differentiation of adenocarcinoma cells that may be observed in pleural fluid are striking. There may be well-differentiated cohesive groups of cells with acinar, ductal or papillary configurations that are typical of epithelial origin, or there may be only discrete, single cells without apparent cohesion that may be more difficult to identify as having originated from epithelium. If vacuolation is present, special stains to identify mucus (such as Mucicarmine or Alcian Blue-PAS) may be helpful in demonstrating the presence of secretion, but some vacuoles may be the result of glycogen accumulation or hydropic degeneration and may not stain positively for mucus.

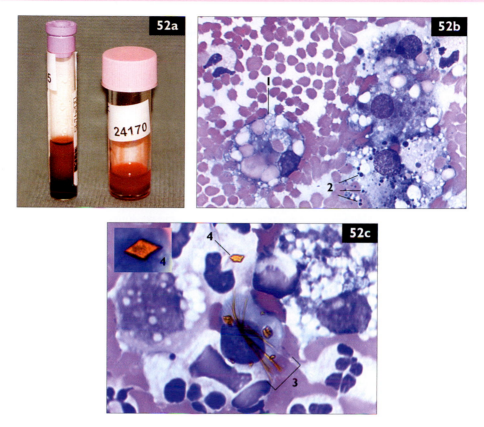

52 Haemorrhagic pleural fluid (**52a**) was aspirated from a nine-year-old Doberman Pinscher that presented with clinical signs of dyspnoea and mild pallor.

a Identify the structures/cells labelled **1, 2, 3** and **4** (**52b, c**) (Wright–Giemsa, ×100 oil), and state their significance.

b Which of the findings indicate chronic haemorrhage?

c Which special stain would you request to confirm that haemosiderin (labelled **2**) from blood breakdown pigment is present and contains iron?

d List three common causes of haemorrhagic effusions and relevant laboratory tests you can use in the investigation of causes of haemorrhagic effusions.

52: Answer

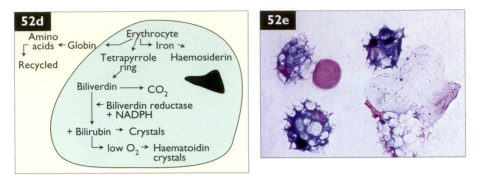

52d — Amino acids ← Globin ← Erythrocyte → Iron → Haemosiderin; Tetrapyrrole ring; Biliverdin → CO₂; Biliverdin reductase + NADPH; + Bilirubin → Crystals; low O₂ → Haematoidin crystals; Recycled

52e

52 a 1 = erythrophagocytosis (can occur in transit or *in situ*); **2** = haemosiderin (is a more stable but less available form of iron, composed of ferritin and denatured ferritin protein in lysosomes); **3** = bilirubin crystals (these are the primary end product of haem degradation in most mammals, by the conversion of biliverdin to bilirubin by biliverdin reductase); **4** = haematoidin crystals (these are an insoluble crystalline form of bilirubin, chemically identical to bilirubin). Sometimes referred to as 'tissue bilirubin', haematoidin forms when oxygen tension is low (hypoxic conditions). Haem oxygenase, the enzyme that cleaves the tetrapyrrole haem ring once the amino acids and iron are liberated, uses molecular oxygen and NADPH. Therefore, haematoidin is often observed with tissue or intracavity haemorrhage in mammals (see **52d** for a flow diagram of RBC breakdown within a macrophage).

b 2, 3, and **4.** Not **1,** because it can occur in transit.

c Perl's Prussian Blue stain: stains iron blue to black (**52e**) (Perl's Prussian Blue, ×100 oil). The blue to blue-black staining within macrophages indicates the presence of iron.

d Considerations for haemorrhagic effusions should include: coagulopathy (test APTT and PT from clotting cascade); trauma (clinical history and external signs); neoplasia (pH strip – a pH >7.0 is supportive of neoplasia and a pH <7.0 is more commonly associated with a benign cause).

Note: The use of pH to help differentiate benign from neoplastic effusions is controversial. Measurements should be done on freshly collected fluid. Other differential diagnoses that should be considered with haemorrhagic effusions include vascular rupture or compromise, organ torsion, rodenticide toxicity or iatrogenic contamination. In some cases, iatrogenic contamination may be easily differentiated from true haemorrhage but in others it may be difficult or impossible to differentiate unless features supporting haemorrhage, such as presented in this case, are present. Iatrogenic contamination is supported by a change from clear or yellow to bloody as the specimen is aspirated. The presence of platelets in the smears supports iatrogenic contamination or very recent haemorrhage, since they disappear rapidly from fluids containing blood. In fluids containing true haemorrhage the sample seldom clots and platelets are rarely seen unless very recent haemorrhage has occurred. In fluid specimens fixed in 40–50% ethanol or with 10% formalin for Papanicolaou preparations immediately after collection, the presence of erythrophagocytosis supports recent haemorrhage since fixation prevents phagocytosis of erythrocytes during specimen transport.

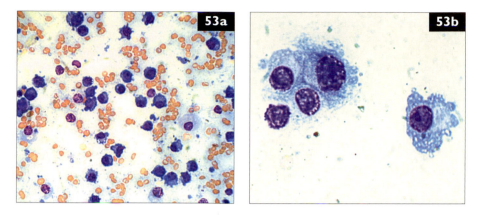

53 A ten-year-old neutered male Cocker Spaniel presented with a mass at the entrance to the external ear canal.
a Describe the cells shown in these smears (53a, b) (Wright–Giemsa, ×50 oil and ×100 oil, respectively).
b What is your interpretation, and what are the differential diagnoses?
c What is the expected biological behaviour?

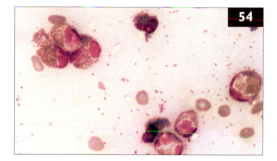

54 An eight-year-old DLH cat presents with a flat, ulcerated lesion on the upper lip measuring approximately 2 cm × 0.5 cm. Dried blood covers part of the lesion and it is slightly raised. Examination of the mouth reveals an ulcerative lesion on the caudodorsal aspect of the tongue. Fine needle aspiration of the lesion is performed with care and smears are prepared (54) (Wright's, ×100 oil).
a What is your diagnosis?
b What therapy is recommended?

53 a There are moderate numbers of erythrocytes and nucleated cells. The nucleated cells are discrete 'round cells' and sometimes occur in small, loosely associated groups. They have oval nuclei that vary from central to eccentric. The chromatin is clumped and sometimes distributed in clumps around the periphery of the nuclear membrane ('clock-face' configuration). Occasionally, a nucleolus is present. The cytoloplasm is moderate and varies from oval to irregularly shaped. In some cells there is a moderately to deeply basophilic cytoplasmic periphery, and an area of more pale staining or clearing can be seen adjacent to the nucleus.
b The cytological features are consistent with a round cell tumour. The features do not support histicytoma, transmissible venereal tumour or mast cell tumour. The features are suggestive of lymphoid origin with plasmacytic differentiation. The primary consideration should be cutaneous plasmacytoma.
c Cutaneous plasmacytomas usually occur in aged dogs. Cocker Spaniels may be predisposed. They are usually solitary and are most commonly seen on the digits, lips and ears. The neoplastic cells may vary from well-differentiated to extremely pleomorphic. Amyloid may be seen in approximately 10% of these tumours and it has been suggested that plasmacytomas containing amyloid are more likely to recur after surgery. The treatment of choice is surgical removal. Local recurrence and metastasis are rare with complete removal.

54 a The location of the lesion, the concurrent presence of a similar lesion on the tongue and the cytological observations are compatible with an indolent ulcer. This lesion forms part of the eosinophilic granuloma complex (EGC). Other lesions included in this complex include the eosinophilic granuloma or linear granuloma and eosinophilic plaque, all cutaneous or mucocutaneous lesions found in cats. There is a possible link to allergens with these lesions, and for this reason the environment should be checked for possible allergens (e.g. flea bite sensitivity, food allergy and/or atopy).
b Corticosteroid therapy is recommended. Long-acting corticosteroid injections (methylprednisolone) (once every 2 weeks for 3 injections or until resolution of lesions if this occurs earlier). Some lesions are refractory to this treatment and require more aggressive therapy (e.g. combination with antihistamine treatment, antibiotic therapy). Recurrence may warrant repeating the series of injections. Refractoriness or recurrence is an indication to examine the possibility of food allergies, as these tend to be associated with refractory EGC lesions.
Note: The cytological finding of mixed inflammation, including eosinophils, is not specific for eosinophilic plaque/granuloma complex but, in conjunction with the clinical appearance of the lesion, supports this diagnosis. Differential diagnoses for this type of inflammation include reactions to foreign bodies or insect, spider or other types of bite wounds, fungal infections or fly irritation. Aspirates are recommended rather than impression smears from the surface of lesions since this type of inflammation may be seen with ulcerated skin and/or mucocutaneous tumours, and impression smears may not provide the variety of cells that occur deeper in the tissue.

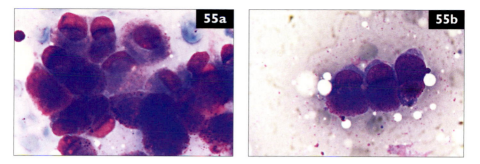

55 Bone marrow aspiration is performed on a dog with a thrombocytopenia.
a Describe the cells represented in these smears (**55a, b**) (both May–Grünwald–Giemsa, ×100 oil).
b What is your diagnosis, and what are the differential diagnoses?

56 Quality assurance programmes are required to monitor, evaluate and improve laboratory performances. Guidelines for quality assurance programmes in veterinary cytology have been provided by the ASVCP Committee on Quality Assurance and Standards. What are the principles of quality assurance in veterinary cytology, and how can diagnostic accuracy be determined in veterinary cytology?

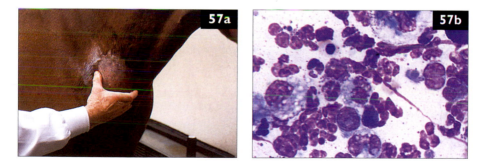

57 An FNA was collected from a firm, painless mass on the shoulder of a Thoroughbred gelding (**57a**).
a What cells are present in this smear (**57b**) (Wright–Giemsa, ×100 oil)?
b What is your diagnosis?

61

55 a There are clusters of bizarre cells in a poorly cellular and haemorrhagic sample. The cells have a small size, more or less adjacent borders, and a clearly polarized aspect with a basal, oval or crescent shaped nucleus and a round, unipolar basophilic cytoplasm containing numerous purple granules. In **55b** the three cells have a palisading appearance.
b Diagnosis: bone marrow metastasis from a pancreatic adenocarcinoma (purple cytoplasm granules probably correspond to zymogen granules). Differential diagnoses: other adenocarcinoma; myeloma because of the confusing plasma cell aspect; mast cell tumour because of the purple granules, but the polarized aspect of the cells and the cohesive sheets argue against a mast cell tumour.

56 Laboratory performance and quality of the results can be affected by preanalytical, analytical and postanalytical factors. Documentation of specific policies, monitoring and corrective actions should be established for all areas of the laboratory by quality assurance programmes. In veterinary cytology, specimen collection, handling, delivery and identification are preanalytical factors that should be addressed and standardized. The cytologist has an essential role in offering educational support to clients and in reducing the number of inadequate specimens submitted.

Standard preparations, fixation and staining procedures of specimens are analytical factors addressed by internal nonstatistical quality control programmes; these can vary between individual laboratories according to the techniques used and cytologist preferences. Diagnostic accuracy should be determined through follow-up procedures. This consists of comparison of findings with histological or additional cytological specimens, information from the animal and other diagnostic tests in order to assess correlation of the results. When discrepancies between results are noted, specimen review is indicated to determine if there are features that have been overlooked or misinterpreted.

Finally, the accuracy of results can be affected by postanalytical factors. A standard format for the reports, which should be easily interpretable and with appropriate explanations, is the cytologist's responsibility. Attribution of the interpretation to the correct animal and reporting of the results to the correct clinician in a timely manner are other aspects of the postanalytic process.

57 a A mixed cell population, mainly of neutrophils, with many reactive macrophages, disrupted eosinophils (in other fields) and a mast cell (top right). Microorganisms are not seen.
b Chronic, active and eosinophilic sterile inflammation.
Note: Eosinophils may be seen as a part of a nonspecific inflammatory response, but considerations should include the possibility of a reaction to a foreign body, migrating parasite, fungal or yeast infection, habronemiasis, or irritation due to fly bites or ulceration (not seen in this case). Eosinophilic inflammation in the horse is a relatively common finding and a specific underlying cause may not always be apparent.

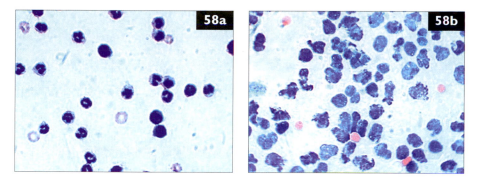

58 A pleural fluid specimen is collected from a ten-year-old entire female Siamese-cross cat, and smears prepared.

a Describe the features shown (58a, b) (Wright–Giemsa, both ×100 oil).

b Why is there a difference in the appearance of these two preparations?

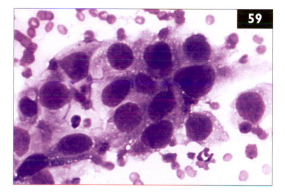

59 A nine-year-old female Samoyed presents with dysuria and haematuria. Urinalysis of a free-catch sample reveals pyuria, haematuria, bacteriuria and numerous, variably sized transitional cells demonstrating multinucleation and anisokaryosis. Palpation and contrast cystography reveal a poorly defined mass in the trigone area of the bladder. Slides are prepared from material obtained following ultrasound-guided fine needle aspiration (59) (Wright's, ×100 oil).

a What is the most likely diagnosis?

b What treatment(s) can be recommended?

58 a There is a slight protein background with a few erythrocytes and many nondegenerated neutrophils in **58a**. There are a few erythrocytes and many poorly preserved cells with swollen nuclei that are rounding up in **58b**. A few cells show slight indentation in the nuclei. These cells are difficult or impossible to identify, but are consistent with neutrophils.

b The difference in appearance is due to the effects of transport. **58a** is from a slide prepared from a freshly collected specimen. **58b** is from the same specimen; it was unfixed and had overnight delivery to the laboratory prior to preparation of the smear. This illustrates the need to prepare a smear from a freshly collected specimen. Fixation (with 10% buffered formalin or 40% ethanol) would help preserve morphology but requires staining with stains other than the commonly available Romanowsky stains, such as Pollack's Trichrome or a Papanicolaou stain.

59 a The signalment, history, palpation, imaging and cytological observations are most compatible with transitional cell carcinoma, the most common bladder neoplasm in the dog. Cytological key features include: cells that are found singly or in aggregates, marked anisocytosis and anisokaryosis, presence of cytoplasmic vacuoles in some cells, variable cytoplasmic basophilia and nuclear:cytoplasmic ratios.

b Currently, surgery is the preferred treatment in dogs in cases in which metastasis is absent, with median survival times of up to one year if there is no concurrent involvement of the urethra and if complete excision is possible. Chemotherapeutic agents such as cisplatin or carboplatin have been reported to be of benefit in some cases. Piroxicam administration may be helpful for palliative treatment.

Note: Transitional cell carcinoma may be a difficult diagnosis in cases with extensive haemorrhage and/or inflammation and atypical cells associated with irritation and whose features may mimic malignancy. Degeneration of cells may further complicate evaluation for features of malignancy.

Collection of specimens other than the first urine in the morning may be of benefit in obtaining cells with less degeneration. Gentle catheter trauma in the area of a mass that has been demonstrated by radiography and/or ultrasound may be helpful in obtaining large numbers of cells. Fixation immediately in an approximately equal volume of cold 40–50% ethanol or addition of two drops of 10% buffered formalin per ml of specimen followed by refrigeration prior to submission to the laboratory is helpful in preserving cellular morphology when Papanicolaou staining is available. If Papanicolaou staining is not available and Romanowsky staining is, preparation of an air-dried smear from sediment from a freshly collected specimen is recommended. Refrigeration of the urine specimen is of benefit in preserving cellular morphology if the specimen cannot be processed immediately.

A relatively new test that is complementary to cytological evaluation and is helpful in providing additional information regarding the likelihood of urinary tract neoplasia is the V-BTA test.

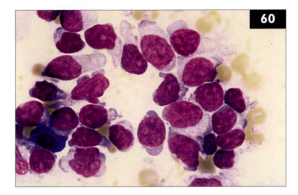

60 An FNA is collected from a canine lymph node.
a Describe the cells shown in this photomicrograph (**60**) (May–Grünwald–Giemsa, ×100 oil).
b What is your diagnosis, and what are the differential diagnoses?

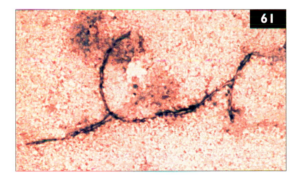

61 A 13-year old neutered male DSH cat presents with inspiratory dyspnoea, frequent sneezing, congestion, weight loss and partial anorexia of three months' duration. Physical examination reveals bilateral mucopurulent nasal discharge. Amoxicillin/clavulanic acid has been administered unsuccessfully. Vaccinations are up-to-date and the cat is free roaming. A smear is prepared from a nasal flush (**61**) (Wright's, ×40). Cranial radiographs do not reveal any osteolytic lesions or evidence of a mass.
a What is your diagnosis based on cytological observation?
b What other diagnostic tests can be performed to support this diagnosis?
c What treatment can be recommended?

60 a An homogeneous population of small lymphoid cells with repeated atypias: extended, clear cytoplasm with a frequent 'hand mirror' aspect and a small clear nucleolus in the nucleus. The chromatin remains more or less clumped.
b Diagnosis: small clear cell lymphoma (T-zone lymphoma) (T-cell phenotype: CD3+, CD4+, CD79a-). Differential diagnosis: none.
Note: The 'hand mirror' aspect refers to the elongation of cytoplasm projecting from some of the lymphoid cells. The projection gives the cell the outline of a hand mirror, with the face of the mirror represented by the nucleus and the handle represented by the cytoplasmic projection.

61 a The microphotograph illustrates a hyphal structure compatible with *Aspergillus* species. Nasal aspergillosis is therefore the likely diagnosis. This infection is more common in dogs than in cats, particularly long-nosed breeds (e.g. Collies).
b Rhinoscopy can reveal atrophy of turbinates and the presence of white or grey plaques. Histological examination, like cytology, can demonstrate fungal hyphae; these are nonpigmented, segmented and branching structures; fungal culture can be performed on material obtained from a nasal flush or tissue sampling during rhinoscopy. Serology for detection of antibodies against *Aspergillus* species is a complementary diagnostic tool but less useful, as false positives do occur. A positive test supports prior exposure to the organism but does not confirm current infection. A negative antibody test does not rule out the possibility of *Aspergillus* infection. Radiographic examination may reveal nonspecific osteolytic lesions that may also be observed with neoplasia. It should be noted that for cytological examination, material obtained via a nasal flush or biopsy is preferred to nasal secretions, which may not contain the organism.
c Oral fluconazole or itraconazole can be administered; topical infusion of an antifungal drug such as clotrimazole has been shown to be effective in dogs, and may clear infections more successfully than systemic therapy.
Note: *Aspergillus* organisms in cytological preparations are usually observed as uniform, septate hyphae of 3–6 microns in width with 45-degree angle (dichotomous) branching. A differential diagnosis is phycomycosis, but these fungi are rarely septate. The presence of septate, branching hyphae in a nasal cytological preparation is strongly supportive of aspergillosis. Definitive diagnosis is by evaluation of reproductive structures, which are seldom seen in cytological specimens but can be identified in preparations of fungal cultures.

Nasal flushings can be very frustrating because they may reflect nonspecific inflammation and may not contain diagnostic features. Client education regarding the possibility of a nonrepresentative specimen and the possible need to progress to nasal biopsy is recommended. Nasal biopsy specimens taken from multiple locations may be needed and aggressive sampling is recommended to obtain specimens that will give the clinician and pathologist confidence in making a diagnosis.

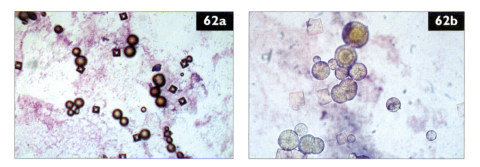

62 An eight-year-old Thoroughbred-cross gelding presented with suspected polyuria and polydipsia. A urine sample is collected and smears prepared.
a What are the structures shown (62a, b) (Wright–Giemsa, ×50 oil and ×100 oil, respectively)?
b What is the significance of these findings?
c What is your interpretation?

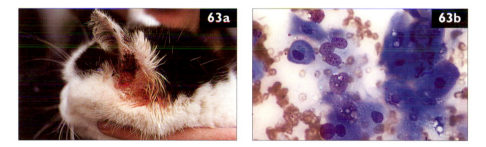

63 A cat presents with ulceration and bleeding from the ear and side of the face (63a). An FNA is collected and a smear made (63b) (Wright–Giemsa, ×100 oil).
a What cells are present?
b What is your diagnosis?

64 An FNA is collected from a canine lymph node.
a Describe the cells represented in this photomicrograph (64) (May–Grünwald–Giemsa, ×100 oil).
b What is your diagnosis, and what are the differential diagnoses?

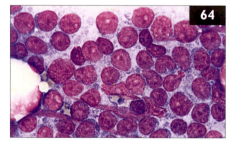

62 a Calcium carbonate and calcium oxalate dihydrate crystals. The calcium carbonate crystals are the rounded structures. Radiating striations from the central core are visible in many crystals in the high-magnification figure. The rectangular/square crystals with a central cross (like an envelope) are the calcium oxalate dihydrate crystals.
b The calcium carbonate crystals are within normal limits in equine urine. Horses absorb calcium from the intestinal tract and eliminate excess calcium in the urine. The calcium oxalate dihydrate crystals may also be within normal limits and tend to appear when the animal is eating oxalate-containing plants.
c The interpretation of this specimen is: no abnormality detected. The findings are within normal limits.

63 a Apart from many RBCs and clumps of neutrophils and cell debris, there is a very pleomorphic population of squamous epithelial cells. These vary from almost spindloid cells with indefinite edges, to clearly squamous cells. Some have deeply basophilic cytoplasm with perinuclear vacuolation. There is some multinucleation, nuclear chromatin clumping and anisokaryosis. The cells are considered to be neoplastic squamous epithelial cells.
b Squamous cell carcinoma, a common finding in encrusted lesions on the pinnae and face of cats.
Note: Squamous cell carcinoma can vary from a very well-differentiated to a very anaplastic, poorly differentiated tumour. Cytological features of squamous differentiation that may be found include keratinization, keratin 'pearls', intercellular bridges (cytoplasmic projections between adjacent cells) and/or polygonal cell shape with low nuclear:cytoplasmic ratio. The presence of keratin precursors within squamous epithelial cells may be heralded by 'baby blue' cytoplasmic staining with Romanowsky stains or the presence of orangophilia with Papanicolaou stain. In more anaplastic tumours the features that aid in recognition of squamous epithelial origin may be focal, infrequent or absent. Squamous epithelial cells with spindloid or elongated appearance are also known as 'tadpole cells'. In well-differentiated tumours, nuclear features supportive of malignancy may be few, but the number of cells, location, smear pattern and presence of an abnormal proliferation provide the background for interpretation of malignancy. Some squamous cell carcinomas may be ulcerated and include abundant neutrophilic and/or eosinophilic inflammation; the presence of inflammation does not ever rule out the possibility of concurrent neoplasia.

64 a An homogeneous population of small cells characterized by a prominent nucleolus that stands up among the clumped chromatin.
b Diagnosis: prolymphocytic lymphoma (B-cell phenotype: CD79a+, CD3-). Differential diagnoses: prolymphocytic T-cell lymphoma, which exhibits the same morphology. The absence of normal residual plasma cells in the background argues for a B-cell lymphoma.

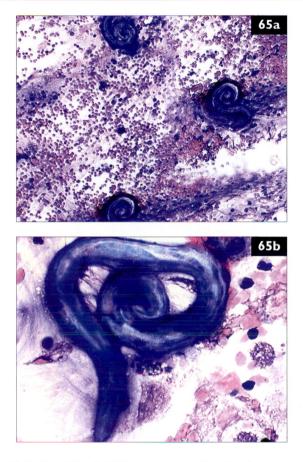

65 A one-year-old Staffordshire Bull Terrier presented with a hard dry cough that had progressed to haemoptysis. Thoracic radiographs revealed a miliary interstitial pattern. A bronchoalveolar lavage was performed and smears made from the wash obtained.

a How would you describe the wash, and what are the coiled structures (**65a**) (Wright–Giemsa, ×50 oil)?

b At high magnification these larvae demonstrate kinked tails (**65b**) (Wright–Giemsa, ×100 oil). What is the most likely differential in dogs? If similar larvae were identified in cats, what is the most likely differential?

c Is an intermediate host required in the life cycle of *Filaroides* species? If so, name the species, and if not, comment why.

d How would you confirm the diagnosis?

65 a Mixed (macrophages and neutrophils) inflammation (pneumonia) with evidence of chronic (resolving) active haemorrhage. The kinetics of the haemorrhage can be determined due to the presence of platelets (active) and haemosiderin (chronic) (seen in other fields of view). The coiled structures are first-stage parasitic larvae <200 microns in length.
b *Filaroides* species (*Oslerus osleri* and *F. hirthi*) in a dog; *Aleurostrongylus abstrusus* in a cat.
c No intermediate host is required, since *Filaroides* species are directly infective as first-stage larvae, and development through all five stages is completed in the lung tissue of the dog. Infection is acquired through the ingestion of regurgitated stomach contents, lung tissue or faeces of infected dogs. Autoinfection can thus worsen the worm burden within an animal.
d Faecal specimens, using zinc sulphate flotation or Baermann technique to identify the larvae.
Note: Filaroid worms in dogs have been reported in many countries, including the USA, UK, South Africa, New Zealand, France and Australia. They vary in length from 5 to 15 mm. If endoscopy is used for collection of a respiratory cytology specimen and evaluation of the respiratory tract, nodules in the area of the distal trachea or area of bifurcation of the major bronchi are classically associated with O. osleri. *F. hirthi* occurs in the lung parenchyma. The bitch may transfer larvae in its saliva to puppies. Following ingestion, larvae are carried by blood to the lungs.

A. vasorum is a relatively common lungworm in the UK. It has a snail intermediate host and may present with coagulopathy, particularly bleeding into the lung. It is reported to be common in racing Greyhounds, but may be seen in a variety of working and pet dogs.

Cytology is best for diagnosis of *F. hirthi*, but low-grade infections may not produce sufficient larvae to be detected. Either zinc sulphate flotation or a Baermann technique may be useful in demonstrating larvae. Fenbendazole (50 mg/kg p/o q24h for 14 days) or albendazole (50 mg/kg p/o q12h for 5 days and repeated in 21 days) have been reported to be effective treatments for *F. hirthi*.

Angiostrongylus abstrusus has been reported in cats in the USA, Europe and Australia. Eggs in alveoli hatch into larvae, which may be coughed up, swallowed and passed in the faeces. Snails or slugs are intermediate hosts and frogs, lizards, birds or rodents may transport encysted larvae, and, if a snail, slug or transport host is eaten, the larvae migrate from the stomach to the lungs. Prevalence of infection is reported to be high, but clinical signs are seldom reported. When present, these may include coughing, dyspnoea, wasting and/or pulmonary rales.

Inflammation with lungworm infection can be extremely variable. Live worms may generate little inflammation. Dead or dying worms are associated with a more obvious inflammatory reaction that may include increased eosinophils and macrophages. *Filaroides* larvae have been reported to be more likely to result in neutrophilic inflammation than eosinophilic inflammation.

66 An eight-year-old DSH cat presented with a six-month history of weight loss and lethargy. Physical examination revealed moderate to severe emaciation. The cat had a poor coat and was slightly icteric. Slight dehydration was present. A mass was palpated in the mid-cranial abdomen. Radiographs revealed a soft tissue superimposition in the area of the stomach/liver. Abnormal biochemistry

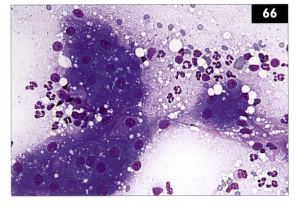

findings were: AST = 177 U/l (ref. = 2–36 U/l); ALT = 557 U/l (ref. = 6–88 U/l); ALP = 201 U/l (ref. = 2–43 U/l); bilirubin = 68 µmol/l (ref. = 0–3.4 µmol/l); TP = 95 g/l (ref. = 65–86 g/l). A smear was made from an FNA of the liver (66) (Wright–Giemsa, ×25).

a Describe the cytological findings, and give your cytological interpretation.
b Briefly discuss the condition.
c How is this condition different from the nonsuppurative cholangiohepatitis seen in cats?

67 A 16-week-old female Husky-cross presented for persistent diarrhoea. A faecal smear was prepared.

a Describe the organisms seen (67) (Gram's, ×100 oil).
b Are the spore-forming gram-positive rods likely to be *Clostridium perfringens*?

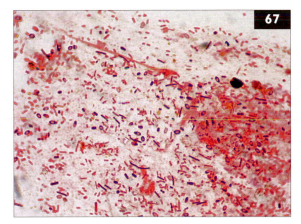

66 a The smear contains many hepatocytes with distinct cytoplasmic vacuoles suggestive of lipid. Large numbers of neutrophils are noted around the hepatocytes and in the background. Neutrophil numbers are significantly increased compared with what would be expected from the peripheral blood contamination alone. The cytological interpretation is suppurative cholangiohepatitis and mild vacuolar degeneration suggestive of lipid.

b Approximately 20% of cats with liver disease are diagnosed with cholangiohepatitis. Cholangiohepatitis can be suppurative, with neutrophils present in the periportal areas and parenchyma. The aetiology is unknown, although ascending bacterial infection from the intestine is suspected. There is no breed or gender predilection for cholangiohepatitis, but most cats are middle aged to older. In addition to liver biopsy, culture of hepatic tissue as well as gastrointestinal biopsies may be helpful in identifying the cause of the inflammation.

c Nonsuppurative cholangiohepatitis is more common than suppurative hepatitis in the cat. The nonsuppurative form is thought to be a progression from the suppurative form. An immune-mediated component has been suggested for this form. Biliary cirrhosis may result from the chronic form.

Note: Marked blood contamination in an animal with an elevated WBC count may contribute to the presence of leukocytes in a liver aspirate. If neutrophils are intimately associated with the hepatocytes, this lends support to an interpretation of hepatitis. In some cases with nodular hyperplasia of the liver, there may be infiltration of neutrophils and lymphocytes that may not be related to hepatitis. The possibility of a concurrent inflammatory condition may be considered. The absence of increased inflammatory cells in a liver aspirate does not rule out the possibility of hepatitis or cholangiohepatitis, particularly if there is a focal distribution. The old adage regarding absence of findings in a cytological specimen applies here: 'The absence of evidence is not evidence of absence'. Cytological aspirates may be very useful in evaluation of the liver, but biopsy may be required for definitive diagnosis of many conditions.

67 a There is a well-mixed population of gram-negative rods, gram-positive rods and small cocci and gram-positive, rounded rods with central spores that often distend the sporangium (the middle of the bacteria).

b No. *Clostridium perfringens* are gram-positive spore-forming rods, but they are classically square-ended and the central spore does not distend the sporangium. These are more likely to be *Bacillus* species, a huge group of aerobic gram-positive spore-formers that are common in the environment. Many have rapid generation times and can overgrow in diarrhoeic stool; they may be able to thrive where other organisms are purged by the rapid transit. The similarities between these two genera, cytologically, may contribute to the controversy regarding *C. perfringens*' role in diarrhoea.

Note: Whenever gram-positive, spore-forming rods are seen in a faecal smear and *Clostridium perfringens* or *Bacillus* species is suspected, confirmation by culture and/or endotoxin assay should be considered in order to provide a definitive diagnosis.

68 Abdominal fluid is aspirated from a 14-year-old neutered male Labrador-cross dog. Analysis reveals: TP = 10 g/l; erythrocytes = 10×10^9/l; NCC = 0.4×10^9/l. A cytospin preparation is prepared and smears made.
a What cell types are seen (68) (Wright–Giemsa, ×100 oil)?
b How would you classify this fluid?
c What considerations/comments would you have regarding this classification?

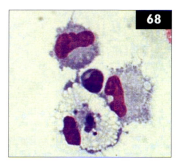

69 A four-year-old Giant Schnauzer presents for a routine check-up prior to elective dental surgery. Physical examination reveals enlarged submandibular lymph nodes. The owner reports no clinical signs. The dog lives in close proximity to a river. A smear is made from an FNA of the enlarged lymph nodes.
a The background contains a dense population of inflammatory cells.

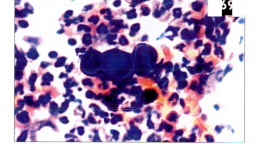

Identify the structures in the centre of the smear (69) (Wright's, ×50 oil).
b What is your diagnosis?
c The dog exhibits no clinical signs other than the enlarged submandibular lymph nodes. No other lymph nodes appear enlarged. What therapy would you recommend?

70 An FNA was taken from a mass in the jugular groove of a 12-year-old cat. The history was of weight loss, with an elevated heart rate. Total T4 was 14 nmol/l (ref. = 10–55 nmol/l).
a Describe the cells seen in this smear (70) (Wright–Giemsa, ×100 oil).
b What is the likely diagnosis?

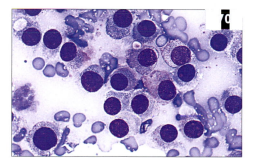

68 a A small lymphocyte (centre), a monocyte (top) and two macrophages. There was a low density of nucleated cells in the cytospin, a finding that would be expected based on the NCC.
b A transudate.
c Transudates are classically associated with hypoproteinaemia/hypoalbuminaemia. Albumin levels are usually <15–18 g/l before effusion will form due to hypoalbuminaemina alone. Transudates may also be seen with early cardiac insufficiency or other noninflammatory conditions. In this case, evaluation of serum chemistry for TP and albumin should be recommended as an initial step.

69 a Yeast-like forms of the genus *Blastomyces*, a broad-based budding yeast that is basophilic and possesses a blue capsule with routine (Romanowsky) stains.
b Blastomycosis. This infection most commonly manifests as a respiratory, ocular or cutaneous infection. Despite the absence of clinical signs, a thorough ocular examination should be done to determine whether uveitis is present; chest radiographs would enable detection of pulmonary disease; also, close examination of the skin may reveal lesions. Blastomycosis is more frequent in animals in close proximity to a body of water, as well as in hunting or sporting breeds.
c Oral administration of the antimycotic drug itraconazole for 60–90 days is the preferred treatment. Alternative drugs include the more toxic, less effective but cheaper drug ketoconazole or intravenously administered amphotericin-B.

70 a The smear shows many erythrocytes and many small mature lymphocytes. A few larger lymphocytes and macrophages are seen. There are groups of cells with features of malignancy and squamous differentiation. These cells have large oval nuclei, often with macronucleoli of varying shapes, often angular, and moderate to abundant cytoplasm that has crisply defined edges and appears pale and occasionally slightly vacuolated.
b In spite of the location in the area of the thyroid gland, and the clinical signs that could be consistent with hyperthyroidism, the cytological features are not consistent with thyroid cells. The presence of lymphocytes suggests a lymph node origin, with a metastatic malignancy consistent with squamous cell carcinoma. Further assessment of the patient to locate a primary tumour would be imperative. Evaluation should include examination of the mouth to determine if sublingual squamous cell carcinoma is present and examination of the skin, especially the head and neck, which may drain to the cervical lymph node chain, to determine if cutaneous squamous cell carcinoma is present.

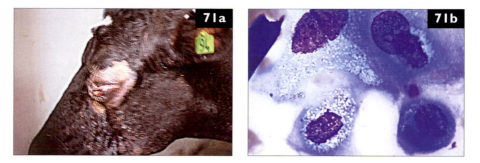

71 A Friesian cow has swollen eyelids, with marked blepharospasm and ocular discharge (71a). An FNA is collected and a smear made (71b) (Wright–Giemsa, ×100 oil).
a What cells are present?
b What is the cytological interpretation?

72 A ten-year-old castrated male Shetland Sheepdog presented with a history of diarrhoea, vomiting, anorexia and lethargy of three days' duration. Physical examination findings included weight loss and dental calculus with mucoid ocular discharge. A cranial abdominal mass was detected on abdominal palpation. Thoracic radiographs were normal. Abdominal radiographs revealed an enlarged liver that displaced the stomach and

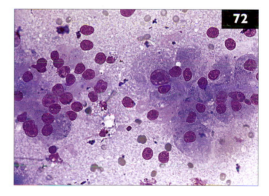

intestines and obstructed the pyloric outflow of the stomach. Ultrasound evaluation of the abdomen showed diffuse involvement of the entire liver. CBC findings included moderate anaemia, leukopenia and thrombocytopenia. The biochemistry profile showed: AST = 8,480 U/l (ref. = 14–38 U/l); ALT = 10,900 U/l (ref. = 10–71 U/l); ALP = 1,476 U/l (ref. = 4–110 U/l); bilirubin = 202 μmol/l (ref. = 0–6.8 μmol/l); BUN = 1.4 mmol/l (ref. = 2.1–9.4 mmol/l); TP = 44 g/l (ref. = 56–75 g/l). A smear was made from an FNA of the liver (72) (Wright–Giemsa, ×25).
a Describe the cytological findings, and give your cytological interpretation.
b Discuss the various forms of this disease seen in the dog.
c Discuss the prognosis for this patient.

71 a The smear contains a lot of neutrophils and cell debris, but there are also clusters of pleomorphic epithelial cells. These vary from benign keratinized mature squames (deep blue structure, top left of **71b**, partially out of the field) to epithelial cells with anisocytosis and basophilic cytoplasm with marked vacuolation. Some of the cells are binucleated, and chromatin clumping and prominent nucleoli are noted. The cell on the bottom right, although nucleated, is deeply stained, suggesting inappropriate keratinization.
b Squamous cell carcinoma. The eyelid is a relatively common site for this tumour in the cow.

72 a The smear contains hepatocytes with moderate to marked malignant features including anisocytosis, anisokaryosis and single to multiple variably sized nucleoli. The chromatin pattern is clumped, with irregular margination. Binucleation and multinucleation are also present. The cytological interpretation is hepatocellular carcinoma.
b Hepatocellular carcinoma is divided into diffuse, nodular and massive forms. Grossly, the diffuse form consists of large areas of the liver infiltrated by nonencapsulated neoplastic tissue; the nodular form consists of multiple discrete nodules of variable size within several lobes; and a massive form consists of a large mass affecting a single liver lobe. Based on the ultrasound findings, the dog in this case likely had a diffuse form. Diffuse and nodular forms in the dog are associated with high metastatic potential (reported to be around 100% and 90%, respectively). The massive forms have relatively less metastatic potential (reported around 35%). Carcinomas may be found in any lobe of the dog liver, although they most commonly occur in the left lateral lobe. Hepatocellular carcinomas usually maintain some degree of hepatocytic differentiation and can often be easily distinguished cytologically from metastatic hepatic neoplasms.
c The prognosis for this patient is poor, based on the high potential for metastatic disease. Metastasis occurs most commonly to the lungs and hepatic lymph nodes. Hepatocellular carcinomas are also known to occasionally metastasize to the heart, spleen, kidney, intestine, brain and ovary via the vascular system. In general, the primary neoplasm is large while the metastases are small. Therefore, the resulting debilitation of the affected animal is usually due to the primary neoplasm and not to the metastatic disease.
Note: The diagnosis of hepatic neoplasia may be difficult, particularly in cases with moderate to severe liver disease. This may result in varying degrees of hepatocellular pleomorphism that may result from degeneration, inflammation and regeneration. A well-differentiated hepatocellular adenoma may resemble normal hepatocytes or have minimal atypia; histological evaluation is usually required for a definitive diagnosis. If hepatic nuclei are stripped of cytoplasm, they may mimic metastatic or infiltrative neoplastic cells because of the presence of their characteristic prominent nucleolus, so care should be taken to evaluate cells with intact cytoplasm. Poorly differentiated hepatocellular carcinomas may be difficult to differentiate from metastatic carcinomas.

73 A ten-year-old neutered female Springer Spaniel presented with a history of coughing. Physical examination and diagnostic imaging revealed the presence of pleural effusion. Thoraco-centesis was performed and 100 ml of slightly yellow fluid was collected (TP = 33 g/l; NCC = 1.1×10^9/l). A cytospin preparation was made from the pleural fluid (73a, b) (Leishman's, ×40 and ×100 oil, respectively). A different area of the cytospin preparation is also shown (73c) (Leishman's, ×100 oil).

a Based on the fluid analysis results, how would you classify this fluid?

b How many different types of nucleated cells can you identify?

c What is your diagnosis?

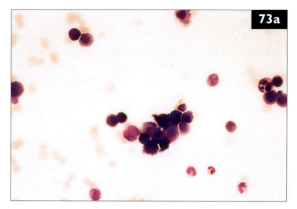

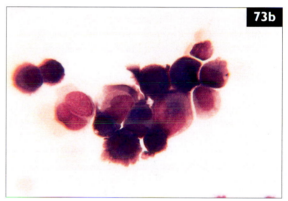

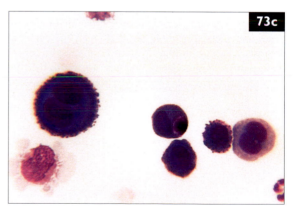

73 a A modified transudate (see Table in answer **31**).

b This is a low cellularity fluid. There are occasional neutrophils and two populations of larger cells. The first population is comprised of cells that show moderate anisocytosis, contain round to oval hyperchromatic nuclei, prominent nucleoli, binucleation, dark basophilic cytoplasm and cytoplasmic fibrils. The second population is comprised of cells that contain oval or indented nuclei with fine chromatin and show binucleation and grey to moderately basophilic cytoplasm. All the cells present are hyperplastic mesothelial cells.

c Modified transudate containing hyperplastic mesothelial cells. The dog was euthanased and a postmortem examination performed. The thorax contained 300 ml of serosanguineous fluid. A nodular mass (4 cm × 3 cm) was found within the mediastinum, close to the heart base. The histological appearance of this mass was suggestive of an ectopic thyroid adenoma.

Note: This case illustrates the range of morphology that may be seen with mesothelial cells. The distinction of hyperplastic versus 'reactive' mesothelial cells has been discussed in human cytological publications but is not usually addressed in veterinary cytology, and the term 'reactive' mesothelium may be more commonly applied to all of the range of changes illustrated in this case. Whether there is any significance in the distinction of hyperplastic versus reactive mesothelial changes is uncertain. The classical appearance of a reactive mesothelial cell is illustrated by the cell to the left in **73c**. This cell has a ruffled or 'sunburst' cytoplasmic border, increased cytoplasmic basophilia and nuclei (two in this cell) that have increased chromatin prominence and small nucleoli.

For readers unfamiliar with the various methods of cytological preparation, the cytospin technique uses a special centrifugal method to concentrate cells in a small area of the slide. This is particularly useful when fluids of low cellularity are obtained and decreases the amount of time that would be needed to view a smear made by the traditional squash preparation or blood smear type methods when low numbers of cells are present. They are particularly useful for cytological preparations from CSF or from pleural or abdominal fluid specimens that may be of low cellularity. Although there may be selective loss of some cell types and slight distortion of others with the cytospin method, it provides a consistent, relatively easy, automated method. Cytospin centrifuges have gone through several generations of improvements and now are within the price range that may be practical for use in veterinary practice. The newest methods of cytological concentration and automated preparation (the best known is Thin-Prep™) currently used in human medicine also concentrate preparations to provide a cell monolayer within a prescribed area on a slide. This technology may become available to veterinary surgeons in the future and provide additional advantages and less cell loss or distortion than that achieved with cytospin techniques.

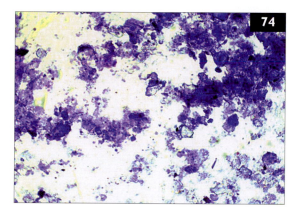

74 A cytospin preparation is made from a CSF sample taken from a two-year-old neutered female King Charles Cavalier Spaniel.
a What is the material shown (74) (Wright–Giemsa, ×50 oil)?
b What are your recommendations based on this finding?

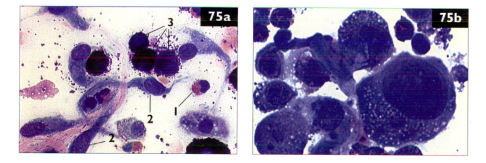

75 An FNA was collected from an eight centimetre, partly ulcerated mass on the hindlimb of an eight-year-old Bull Terrier. The dog was principally presented for melaena. The owner had noted the mass previously, but didn't think it was important since it occasionally increased in size and then decreased in size.
a Identify the cells labelled 1, 2 and 3 (75a) (Wright–Giemsa, ×50 oil). Provide an overall interpretation, and explain the significance of these cells within your interpretation.
b How common is gastroduodenal ulceration in dogs with mast cell tumour?
c What is the prognosis for the tumour represented in 75a compared with 75b (Wright–Giemsa, ×100 oil)?
d Why is it important to aspirate/biopsy the local lymph node in a confirmed mast cell tumour?

74 a Refractile, moderate to deep blue staining, irregularly shaped plates and crystal-like structures. No nucleated cells, erythrocytes or infectious agents are seen. It is suspected to be a contaminant. On further investigation it was found that the specimen had been submitted in a tube with separator beads. When another specimen was added to a tube containing these beads and agitated, the same amorphous, crystalline debris was obtained in the cytological preparation.
b Recommendations for future submissions are to avoid tubes with separator beads or gel. CSF should be submitted in a clean tube to avoid contaminants that may interfere with cytological evaluation.

75 a Mast cell tumour with secondary eosinophil and fibrocyte infiltration. The significance of the individual cells is as follows: **1** = eosinophils: mast cells release eosinophil chemotactic factor, IL3, IL5 and GM-CSF that attract eosinophils. The precise role of eosinophils in mast cell tumours is as yet undetermined. **2** = fibrocytes/fibroblasts: these are often seen in mast cell tumours, since mast cells release chemokines that attract fibrocytes to the tumour location. In a histology section the presence of a fibrocyte component is seen as varying amounts of fibrous connective tissue around the neoplastic mast cells. **3** = neoplastic mast cells.

Mast cell granules contain an impressive array of physiologically active chemical mediators, the two most important being histamine and heparin, the latter imparting the purple-red colour (metachromatic) colour to the granules. Histamine and heparin pose risks in that histamine can result in severe intraoperative hypertension and heparin in some mast cell tumours (usually grade II) can be associated with coagulopathy/haemorrhage.
b 80% of dogs with mast cell tumours develop gastrointestinal ulceration (histamine related).
c Mast cell tumours vary in biological activity but all tumours should be considered to be at least potentially malignant. They can be histologically graded using a system developed by Patnaik (in 1984), based primarily on nuclear morphology, which correlates well with biological behaviour. Classification includes grade I (better prognosis) to grade III (more guarded prognosis). An exception to this guide are mast cell tumours in the perineum and inguinal regions, which tend to be malignant, regardless of grade. **75a** was histologically confirmed as a grade I tumour and **75b** was a grade III tumour. Note how rare the mast cell granules are and the bizarre neoplastic cytological features in the grade III tumour.
d Regional lymph nodes are the site of highest frequency of metastasis.
Note: 75b illustrates well a feature that may be useful in increasing the index of suspicion for mast cell tumour in cases with poor differentiation and few granules. Note the multiple small cytoplasmic vacuoles and the fact that some of these appear to extend across the nucleus. These are hypothesized to represent spaces where granules may have been previously. They differ from vacuoles seen with secretion and adenocarcinoma based on their small size and apparent extension across the nucleus. They do not stain positively for mucus with Mucicarmine or PAS stains.

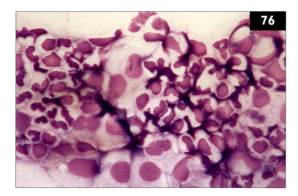

76 A three-year-old gelding was box walking, sweating, stamping and head pressing. A sample of peritoneal fluid was collected and examined immediately. It was turbid and serosanguineous, and had an NCC of $21 \times 10^9/l$ and a TP of 43 g/l. Cells seen in a cytospin preparation of the fluid are shown (**76**) (Wright–Giemsa, ×100 oil).
a What type of fluid is present (fluid classification)?
b What cells are present ?
c What is your diagnosis?

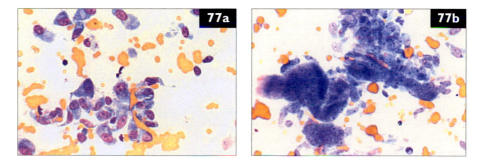

77 A mass on the paw of a nine-year-old neutered male Labrador Retriever is aspirated and smears prepared (**77a, b**) (both Wright–Giemsa, ×50 oil).
a Describe the cells seen.
b What is your cytological interpretation?
c What differential diagnoses would you consider?

76 a The elevated TP and NCC indicate an exudate.
b The cells present are neutrophils (some immature) and macrophages. Although processed immediately, stain take up is very poor and, along with the physical parameters, this suggests an abdominal catastrophe such as intestinal torsion; however, microorganisms and plant material, which would indicate rupture of an intestinal viscus, are absent.
c Peritonitis/possible torsion. Torsion was found on laparotomy.
Note: Reference values for NCCs and classification of effusions in large animals differ from those for small animal specimens. (Guidelines for fluid classification in cows and horses are shown in question **3**.)

77 a There are scattered erythrocytes and many discrete cells with oval, eccentric or basal nuclei, often containing one to several distinct nucleoli. The cytoplasm is moderate and moderately to deeply basophilic, sometimes with a small area of perinuclear clearing (Golgi zone). There are several very large multinucleated cells whose nuclei have the same features as the mononucleated cells. A few cells are elongated and have unipolar or bipolar cytoplasmic extensions.
b A sarcoma.
c Differential diagnoses that should be considered are:
- Giant cell sarcoma of bone (particularly if there is evidence of bone involvement radiographically).
- Malignant fibrous histiocytoma.
- Giant cell sarcoma (variant of fibrosarcoma).
- Disseminated histiocytic sarcoma (also called malignant histiocytosis).
- Plasma cell tumour may be considered based on the features of some of the individual mononuclear cells with eccentric nuclei, basophilic cytoplasm and a small area of perinuclear clearing, but the multinucleated cells and spindle cells that are also part of the picture should lead you away from plasmacytoma and to a tumour of spindle cell/mesenchymal origin.

In this case, there was radiographic evidence of bone involvement. When removed, the tumour could be seen to be arising from the periosteum and small islands of osteoid were also seen. Therefore, the histological diagnosis was giant cell sarcoma of bone.

78 Abdominal fluid is aspirated from a five-year-old entire male Beagle. A smear of the sediment from the fluid is made.
a What features are shown (78) (Wright–Giemsa, ×50 oil)?
b What is the significance of these findings in an abdominal effusion?
c What other features would you like to see to confirm your differential diagnoses?

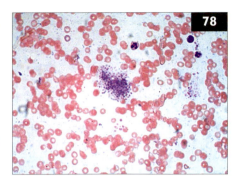

79 Bronchoalveolar lavage is performed on a two-year-old Thoroughbred gelding in racing training presented because of a history of poor performance. A smear of the sediment from the lavage is made.
a What is the structure shown (79) (Wright–Giemsa, ×100 oil)?
b What is the significance of this finding in a respiratory cytology specimen?

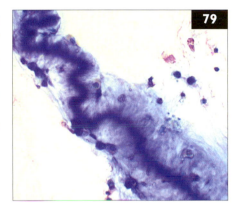

80 A tracheal washing is collected from a six-year-old entire female Fox Terrier with a history of chronic coughing. Radiography shows an interstitial pattern of the lung. A smear is made from sediment from the washing.
a What cell types are shown (80) (Wright–Giemsa, ×100 oil)?
b What is the significance of these cell types?

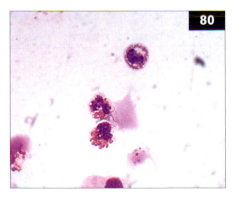

78 a Many erythrocytes, a large clump of platelets (centre) and a few leukocytes.
b The findings are consistent with the presence of fresh blood. Usually, platelets disappear from fresh haemorrhage within 2–4 hours. Their presence supports very recent haemorrhage and/or contamination with blood.
c Other features that would help confirm the following differential diagnoses are:
- Haemorrhage: homogeneous blood stained appearance at the time of collection; if there has been chronic haemorrhage, there may be siderophages.
- Contamination with blood: blood staining appearing during collection; nonhomogeneous blood staining.
- Coagulopathy: abnormal coagulation profile; presence of anaemia.
- Severe congestion, vascular rupture or anomaly: abnormal imaging results, shock, concurrent prediposing disease.

79 a A Curschmann's spiral. It has a dense, central, twisted core, surrounded by a lighter mantle of less dense mucus.
b Curschmann's spirals are a reflection of mucostasis. One end of a strand of mucus is fixed within the airway and the other end is 'free', allowing twisting of the core and accumulation of the less dense mantle of mucus with time. They are a nonspecific finding, but may occur in any condition where there is static mucus. They may contribute to airway narrowing and 'functional' obstruction of airways.

80 a An eosinophilic polymorphonuclear leukocyte (centre), an eosinophilic promyelocyte (bottom) and an eosinophilic myelocyte (top).
b It is not unusual to see immature eosinophils in tracheal washings. The bone marrow does not contain a large eosinophilic polymorphonuclear leukocyte reserve. If there is an increased demand for eosinophils, immature forms may be released from the bone marrow. A mixture of mature and immature forms may be present in many cases. There may or may not be eosinophilia and/or immature eosinophils in the peripheral blood. The finding of immature eosinophils in a tracheal washing should not be interpreted as representing a leukaemic infiltrate unless there is other supporting evidence for leukaemia.

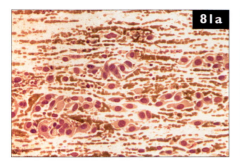

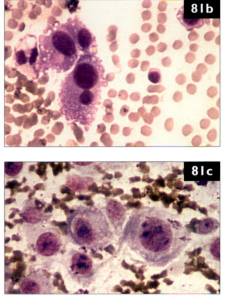

81 A 3.5-year-old entire male Golden Retriever presented with a well-circumscribed, moderately firm, frontal, subcutaneous mass, 4 cm in diameter that had been noted a few weeks previously by its owner. Cranial radiographs revealed a well-circumscribed mass associated with mild osteolysis and bony proliferation in the left frontal sinus. When aspirated, a blood-tinged viscous material was obtained. Several photomicrographs at low-power and high-power magnification illustrate the cytological appearance of this tumour (**81a, b, c**) (Wright's, ×10, ×100 oil and ×100 oil, respectively). What are your differential diagnoses?

82 A six-year-old neutered male Rottweiler presented with a history of stiffness, lethargy and slight bilateral stifle joint effusions. No cranial drawer sign was present. Synovial fluid was collected from

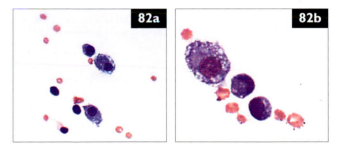

both stifle joints; the fluid from both joints contained similar features. Analysis of the synovial fluid revealed: RBC = <10 × 10^{12}/l; NCC = 3.2 × 10^9/l; TP = 40 g/l; mucin clot test – good; viscosity – good.

a Describe the cell types and features illustrated (**82a, b**) (Wright Giemsa, ×50 oil and ×100 oil, respectively).

b What is your interpretation of this case, and what are your comments?

85

81 The viscous appearance and alignment of RBCs evident at low power suggest a mucinous matrix associated with this neoplasm. The spindle shape of the cells and numerous nuclear features of malignancy suggest a malignant mesenchymal tumour, most likely a myxosarcoma. Nuclear criteria of malignancy include: anisokaryosis, occasional multinucleation (81a, centre), variable nuclear:cytoplasmic ratio, nuclear fragmentation, prominent nucleoli and chromatin smudging. Several other tumours can be characterized by a myxomatous matrix and could be included in a differential diagnosis (e.g. chondrosarcoma, chordoma or myxoid liposarcoma). These tumours can usually be differentiated by their cytological and histological features.

82 a There are a few erythrocytes and a low density of nucleated cells. The mucinous character of the background that is typical of synovial fluid is not apparent in these photomicrographs, but it was present when the glass slide was examined. There are three small darkly stained cells that may be small lymphocytes or synoviocytes in 82a. The cell at the top of this figure is consistent with a small synoviocyte. The other two cells are synoviocytes; these are slightly enlarged with slightly enlarged nuclei and increased chromatin prominence and are not typical of aspirates from normal joints (hyperplastic and hypertrophic synoviocytes). There is slight atypical cytoplasmic vacuolation in the larger synoviocyte toward the top of the picture. 82b shows a higher magnification, with two small dark cells that may be lymphocytes or small synoviocytes and a single slightly hyerplastic and hypertrophic synoviocyte. No neutrophils or infectious agents are visible.
b The cytological features are consistent with slight hyperplasia and hypertrophy of synoviocytes, with slight atypical cytoplasmic vacuolation. The TP is slightly increased, as is the NCC. These findings are nonspecific but are consistent with a response to chronic irritation. These features are not specific for degenerative joint disease/osteoarthritis but are often seen when it is present.

Follow-up radiographs showed moderate osteoarthritic changes associated with both stifle joints. The alterations in synoviocytes may be quite subtle. Recognition of slight changes that may represent deviations from normal requires a careful study of synoviocytes found in normal joints. There is a limited range of changes that synoviocytes undergo in response to irritation or injury. Slight cytoplasmic enlargement, increased chromatin prominence and slight nuclear enlargement are common and indicate increased activity. A variety of conditions may result in this appearance, but degenerative conditions should be included in the differential when this morphology is present. A good smear that is rapidly air-dried, or a Papanicolaou-stained smear, is needed. If the smear is too thick and/or does not air-dry rapidly, the cells may round up and stain darkly, and subtle changes may be difficult or impossible to appreciate.

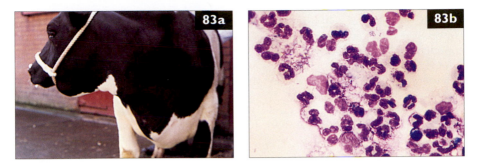

83 Three days after calving, a four-year-old Friesian cow became acutely ill, with brisket and submandibular oedema (83a). She was stiff and grunted with respiration. Peritoneal fluid withdrawn from a site 5 cm cranial and 5 cm medial to the milk well had a TP of 48 g/l and an NCC of 37 ×10⁹/l. A cytospun smear of the peritoneal fluid was prepared (83b) (Wright–Giemsa, ×50 oil).
a What cells are present?
b What is the fluid classification?
c What is your diagnosis?

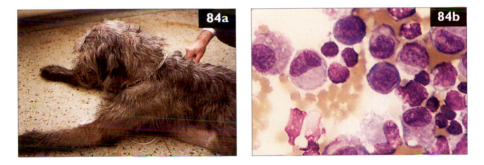

84 A five-year-old male Irish Wolfhound (84a) has become dull and dyspnoeic. Serosanguineous pleural fluid is aspirated (TP = 34 g/l, NCC = 11 × 10⁹/l). A cytospun smear contains the cells shown (84b) (Wright–Giemsa, ×100 oil).
a What cells are present?
b What is the fluid classification?
c What is your diagnosis?

83 a There is a lot of cell disruption and debris, making cell identification difficult. However, the outline of neutrophils is visible in some cases and the disrupted cells are considered to be karyolytic neutrophils. No microorganisms are seen.
b An exudate.
c Acute peritonitis. Given the history and clinical signs, this is suggestive of foreign body reticuloperitonitis.
Note: Reference values for NCCs and classification of effusions in large animals differ from those for small animal specimens. (Guidelines for fluid classification in cows and horses are shown in question **3**.)

84 a The smear is filled with RBCs and a mixed population of nucleated cells. There are many macrophages, small mature lymphocytes, a population of 'round cells' and a few neutrophils and mesothelial cells. The large 'round cells' have basophilic cytoplasm and large, round nuclei, some of which have clumped chromatin. Some have irregularly folded nuclear margins. These cells are considered to be atypical lymphocytes.
b An exudate (see Table in answer **31**).
c These findings are considered to be suspicious for lymphosarcoma. As his condition worsened rapidly, the dog was euthanased and lymphosarcoma was confirmed on postmortem examination.
Note: Various 'round cell' tumours and differential diagnoses for 'round cell tumours' have been illustrated in other cases in this book. This case illustrates 'round cells' considered to be of lymphoid origin. Lymphosarcoma may have a variety of cytological appearances and it may be difficult, in some cases, to differentiate well-differentiated or 'small cell' lymphoma from reactive lymphoid hyperplasia or idiopathic lymphoid reactions. In this case it was not certain whether this was a reactive process, since the larger cells were mixed with a population of small, mature lymphocytes. Demonstration of clonality and/or immunophenotyping for T- and B-cells may have been helpful in this case and in others in which the diagnosis of malignancy is not certain. Evaluation of serial collections can sometimes be useful in demonstrating progression of disease (e.g. persistent atypia and/or increasing proportions of cells with features supportive of malignancy) and, in conjunction with the inability to demonstrate possible underlying causes for a reactive condition, increased confidence in a diagnosis of malignancy may be obtained.

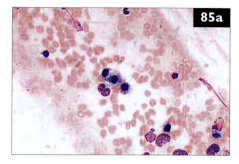

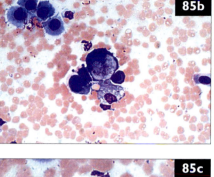

85 A seven-year-old entire male Labrador Retriever presented with pericardial effusion. There was no clinical or radiographic evidence of cardiac disease. Smears were made from the sediment from the pericardial fluid.
a What cell types are shown (85a [Wright–Giemsa, ×50 oil] and 85b, c [Wright–Giemsa, ×100 oil])?
b What is your interpretation of these findings?
c What are your differential diagnoses?

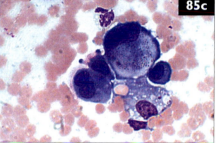

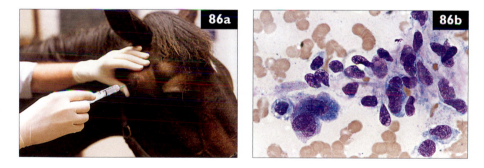

86 A spongy mass is found on the bone lateral and caudal to the eye in a nine-year-old horse from a riding stable. An FNA is collected (86a) and a smear made (86b) (Wright–Giemsa, ×100 oil).
a What cells are present?
b What is your diagnosis?

85 a The cell types include erythrocytes in the background. There are a moderate number of macrophages, with a few lymphocytes and neutrophils. Some of the mononuclear cells contain black pigment granules consistent with melanin. In other fields (see upper left of **85b**), there are reactive mesothelial cells that occur singly and in clusters. The pigment is negative for iron with Perl's Prussian Blue stain.

b This is likely to be a haemorrhagic effusion. An underlying cause for the effusion is not apparent in the cytological preparations. The cells containing melanin are somewhat atypical but are within limits for reactive mesothelial cells or macrophages. Metastatic melanoma may be a consideration when melanin pigment is seen, but it is more likely to be due to hyperpigmentation. Focal pigment deposits may occur on various serosal surfaces. Hyperpigmentation may occur with chronic irritation. Several cases with apparent hyperpigmentation have been seen in pericardial fluid specimens at the author's laboratory. Extended follow up did not indicate the presence of malignant melanoma or other tumours. It may be that melanin is present because of damage to pigmented membrane or pigment deposition.

c Differential diagnoses that should be considered with possible haemorrhagic effusions include:
- Coagulopathy.
- Vascular rupture or anomaly.
- Severe congestion.
- Neoplasia (especially cardiac haemangiosarcoma).

86 a Apart from RBCs, there is a single population of pleomorphic cells. These vary from round to spindle-shaped, and they have basophilic cytoplasm with indefinite boundaries. Nuclei are round to fusiform with clumped chromatin and a single angular nucleolus. The findings are of a mesenchymal cell neoplasm.

b Sarcoma. A fibrosarcoma was confirmed on postmortem examination.

Note: The differential diagnoses that should be considered for spindle cell tumours/mesenchymal tumours in horses include fibroma, fibrosarcoma and equine sarcoid. Other types of mesenchymal tumours are very uncommon. It may be difficult or impossible to differentiate these tumours based on cytological features alone. Consideration of the clinical appearance and location may be helpful, but definitive diagnosis usually requires histological evaluation.

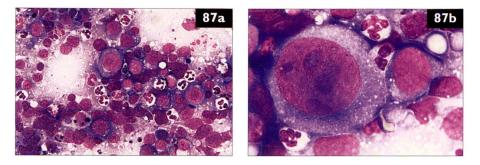

87 An FNA is collected from a canine lymph node.
a Describe the cells shown in these smears (**87a,b**) (May–Grünwald–Giemsa, ×40 and ×100 oil, respectively).
b What is your diagnosis and what are the differential diagnoses?

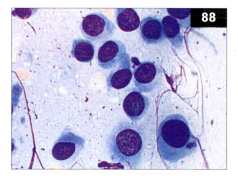

88 An 18-month-old neutered male Dobermann/German Shepherd Dog-cross presented with a well-circumscribed, alopecic, pink mass, approximately 2 cm in diameter, located on the right shoulder. The mass was first noticed five days previously. Fine needle aspiration of both masses is performed and smears are prepared (**88**) (Wright's, ×100).
a What is your diagnosis?
b What treatment do you recommend?

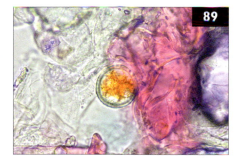

89 A three-year-old spayed female Labrador Retriever presented for hyper-pigmented, lichenified skin on the ventrum, seasonal pruritis, chewing of the feet and inflamed ears. A tape test preparation was obtained from the inflamed ears. No significant *Malasezzia* organisms were found.
a What is the round, yellowish structure (**89**) (Diff-Quik, omitting fixation step, ×40)?
b How might it be related to this dog's problems?

87 a A heterogeneous lymph node population with a mixture of atypical, very large round cells and a heterogeneous inflammatory background is seen in **87a**. At high magnification (**87b**) the round cells have a great variation in size, with a majority of very large cells, a mononuclear aspect with nuclear features of Hodgkin's cell and an extended deeply basophilic cytoplasm, sometimes vacuolated, suggesting plasmablastic differentiation.

b Diagnosis: 'anaplastic' large cell lymphoma (null phenotype: CD79a-, CD3-). Differential diagnosis: atypical immunoblastic lymphoma.

88 a The young age of this animal, the rapid appearance, anterior location and cytological appearance are compatible with a cutaneous histiocytoma, a benign dermal tumour of dogs. The cells are round, discrete cells with well-defined borders. They exhibit moderate anisocytosis and anisokaryosis. Discrete cytoplasmic vacuolation and occasional multinucleation may be noted (not shown). Nuclei are round to ovoid. Nucleoli may vary from inconspicuous to prominent, and may be single or multiple. Lymphocytic infiltration is commonly observed but was not observed in this case.

b This tumour generally regresses spontaneously within a few months such that no therapy is needed unless the mass causes itching or bleeding and discomfort to the animal, or if it does not appear to regress within the anticipated time following observation. A differential diagnosis would include a poorly differentiated mast cell tumour, which may have a similar cytological appearance, especially if a modified Wright's stain or Diff-Quik is used – these may not stain the small number of cytoplasmic metachromatic granules present in poorly differentiated mast cells. However, close examination of a poorly differentiated mast cell tumour specimen, with Wright's or Giemsa staining, will reveal granules in at least a small number of cells. In addition, the cytoplasm will have a different texture, appearing finely granular and more basophilic regardless of whether a modified Wright's or Giemsa stain is used.

Note: Lymphocytes in a regressing tumour and/or presence of neutrophils and bacteria in an ulcerated histiocytoma may sometimes outnumber tumour cells. In these cases it may be difficult to determine if the aspirate represents chronic and active inflammation or pyogranulomatous inflammation, or an inflamed and/or regressing histiocytoma. Histiocytomas with more atypical features are uncommon, but they may be difficult to differentiate from systemic histiocytosis, which may also have cutaneous lesions; these often occur in young dogs.

89 a Some kind of pollen grain. Note the thick cell wall and yellow pigment. There are multiple large, polygonal squames (keratinized, anucleated squamous epithelial cells) in the background.

b With this dog's presentation and the seasonal nature of its problems, allergy to pollens (atopy) is high on the list of diagnostic differentials. The presence of pollen suggests an elevated level in the environment that may be contributing to exacerbation of the allergic condition.

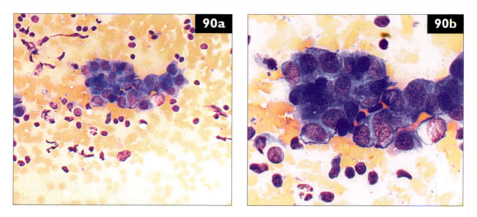

90 An 11-year-old neutered female Miniature Poodle presents with an enlarged axillary lymph node. Smears are made from an aspirate from the node.
a Describe the features illustrated (**90a, b**) (Wright–Giemsa, ×50 oil and ×100 oil, respectively).
b What is your interpretation of these findings?

91 A six-year-old castrated male Miniature Pinscher presented with a history of a perineal skin growth and a palpable abdominal mass. The dog was not feeling well and was constipated. Rectal palpation revealed a palpable mass dorsal to the colon in the area of the sublumbar lymph node. Radiographs revealed sublumbar lymphadenopathy with large amounts of faeces in the colon and a mineralized faecal ball just cranial

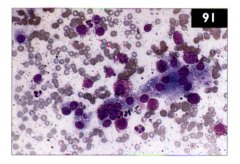

to the stricture formed by the sublumbar lymph node enlargement. A CBC revealed mature neutrophilia, monocytosis and eosinophilia. Abdominal ultrasound findings included multiple small hypoechoic hepatic nodules and mixed echogenic sublumbar masses. Aspirates were obtained from the liver (**91**) (Wright–Giemsa, ×20), the abdominal mass and the perineal mass.
a Describe the cytological appearance, and give your cytological interpretation.
b What do we know about the biological behaviour of these lesions?
c List the treatment options.

90 a There are backgrounds with many erythrocytes and a moderate number of nucleated cells. There are many small, mature lymphocytes in the background, with a few neutrophils. There are scattered clusters and ribbons of cells with apparent intercellular cohesion. These cells have oval nuclei, often containing a single distinct to indistinct nucleolus. There is a relatively high nuclear:cytoplasmic ratio. The cytoplasm varies from scant to moderate and is usually homogeneous and moderately basophilic.
b The cytological features are consistent with carcinoma metastatic to the lymph node. The population of cells is not as expected in a lymph node and it has features supportive of malignancy. The clusters and ribbons, with apparent intercellular cohesion, are supportive of epithelial origin (carcinoma).

Any time an atypical population of cells is present in a lymph node aspirate, metastatic malignancy should be a consideration. In some cases the lymph node may be entirely effaced by the tumour and it may not be possible to decide whether the mass is a primary neoplasm or metastasis to the node. In this case the background, with many small lymphocytes, provides support for the clinical identification of axillary lymph node metastatic malignancy.

91 a The smear contains several hepatocytes with round nuclei and single prominent nucleoli. Some hepatocytes contain blue to green pigment consistent with bile. There are several, individualized round cells present with purple cytoplasmic granules consistent with mast cells. These mast cells have atypical features, which include mild to moderate anisokaryosis, diffuse chromatin pattern and a variable nuclear:cytoplasmic ratio. The cytoplasmic metachromatic granules are present in moderate numbers. One eosinophil is also noted. The cytological interpretation is metastatic mast cell tumour with mild eosinophilic infiltrate.
b The biological behaviour of mast cell tumours depends on the location and cytological differentiation. Mast cell tumours located in the perineal region and at mucocutaneous junctions have a high rate of metastasis, irrespective of the cytological appearance. Mast cell tumour was diagnosed from the perineal mass in this dog. Cutaneous mast cell tumours usually metastasize via lymphatics, but widespread dissemination to bone marrow, liver and/or spleen may eventually occur. In this case, sublumbar lymph node aspirates also contained a metastatic mast cell population.
c There are several therapeutic strategies for treatment of patients with disseminated mast cell tumour. Oral daily prednisone therapy has a long-term success rate of about 25%. Oral lomustine and prednisone therapy has a slightly higher success rate (40% respond). This option entails weekly CBCs to check for bone marrow suppression. A combination of intravenous vinblastin and cyclophosphamide with oral prednisone therapy has also been suggested, but this has possible side-effects including gastrointestinal upset, urinary bladder irritation and bone marrow suppression.

92 A seven-year-old male castrated Rhodesian Ridgeback presented with a history of acute weight loss, anorexia and diarrhoea. Physical examination revealed icterus. Thoracic auscultation and abdominal palpation were within normal limits. Abdominal ultrasound findings included a hypoechoic liver with multiple target lesions, a mottled spleen and a questionable nodular structure in the location of the left lobe of the

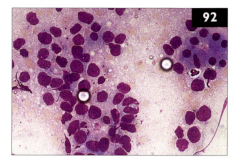

pancreas. Surgical laparotomy was performed. The biochemistry profile was:
AST = 312 U/l (ref. = 14–38 U/l); ALT = 623 U/l (ref. = 10–71 U/l); ALP = 5,955 U/l (ref. = 4–110 U/l); bilirubin = 272 µmol/l (ref. = 0–6.8 µmol/l); BUN = 1.43 mmol/l (ref. = 2.14–9.6 mmol/l); cholesterol = 9.19 mmol/l (ref. = 3.6–8.9 mmol/l); glucose = 0.78 mmol/l (ref. = 4.4–7.0 mmol/l). A liver tissue imprint was prepared (92) (Wright–Giemsa, ×25).
a Describe the cytological findings, and give your cytological interpretation.
b List the differentials for your cytological interpretation.
c What is the prognosis for this patient?

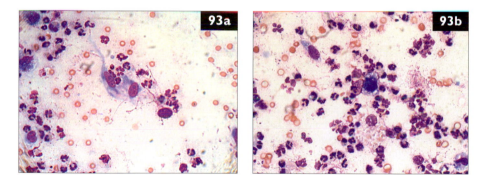

93 A seven-year-old neutered male Jack Russell Terrier presented with an interdigital mass of several weeks' duration. Smears were made from an aspirate of the mass.
a What features are illustrated in these photomicrographs (93a, b) (both Wright–Giemsa, ×50 oil)?
b What is your interpretation of these findings?
c What comments do you have regarding these findings?

92 a The smear contains low numbers of hepatocytes containing abundant cytoplasm with round nuclei and single prominent nucleoli. Several epithelial cells are noted with high nuclear:cytoplasmic ratio and with large round to polygonal nuclei and very pale cytoplasm. These cells have several malignant features including binucleation, anisokaryosis and nuclear moulding. A mitotic figure is also present. The cytological interpretation is carcinoma.
b Differentials include biliary carcinoma or metastatic carcinoma, likely pancreatic in origin. The malignant epithelial cells do not appear to be of hepatocellular origin. Histopathology revealed pancreatic adenocarcinoma with metastasis to the liver.
c The prognosis is grave for patients with metastatic carcinoma in the liver. Pancreatic carcinomas are usually highly aggressive neoplasms. Surgery is not possible due to the diffuse metastatic disease.

93 a There are a few erythrocytes and moderate to high nucleated cellularity. The nucleated cells include many neutrophils, a moderate number of foamy, active macrophages and a few spindle cells. The spindle cells have granular, evenly distributed chromatin and the nuclei contain one to several small but distinct nucleoli. The cytoplasm is wispy and often has bipolar extensions.
b The cytological features are consistent with moderate to marked pyogranulomatous inflammation with spindle cell proliferation, most likely fibroplasia.
c The cytological finding of pyogranulomatous inflammation may be nonspecific, but the possibility of a reaction to a foreign body or penetrating wound of the interdigital area should be considered. This type of inflammation may or may not be easily resolved. The spindle cells are consistent with a proliferative population, most likely a fibroplastic response.

Atypical spindle cells with nucleoli and increased numbers typical of proliferation represent a diagnostic problem for all cytologists. When present in small numbers and accompanied by the type of inflammation found in this specimen, they are most likely due to fibroplasia. However, in some cases, spindle cell proliferations may be difficult to differentiate and it may be difficult or impossible to separate fibroplasia from an actively growing benign tumour or a malignant one. Cellularity, degree of atypia and other concurrent features all have to be considered. In some cases, cytological evaluation can help separate these conditions with a high degree of confidence. In others the differential diagnoses cannot be differentiated on the basis of cytology alone and a biopsy will be needed to determine the definitive diagnosis.

94 A ten-year-old mare arrives at a breeding farm in January without a foal at her side. No previous history is available. A uterine washing is collected to determine the mare's reproductive status.
a Describe the features shown in this smear (**94**) (Papanicolaou, ×100 oil).
b What is your interpretation of these findings?
c What is the significance of these findings?

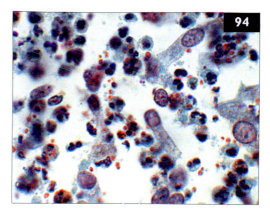

95 An FNA is collected from a canine lymph node.
a Describe the cells shown in this photomicrograph (**95**) (May–Grünwald–Giemsa, ×100 oil).
b What is your diagnosis and what are the differential diagnoses?

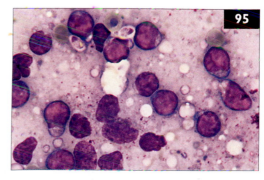

96 A four-year-old Labrador presents with a firm, mildly painful interdigital swelling. An FNA is collected and smears made. These contain neutrophils, plasma cells and the cells shown in **96** (~~~ht–Giemsa, ×100 oil).
~~~ cell in **96**?
~~~osis?

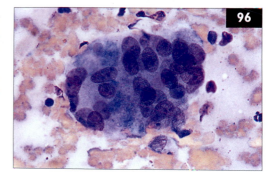

94 a There are a few vacuolated columnar epithelial cells with a few nuclei that have been stripped of cytoplasm. There are a moderate number of macrophages. Within some of the macrophages, and free in the background of the smear, are numerous small, oval organisms that stain red-orange and are consistent with yeast. These are smaller than erythrocytes and do not contain homogeneous haemoglobin within the cell membrane.
b The cytological findings are consistent with uterine yeast infection.
c The significance of this finding is that yeast infection requires antifungal treatment rather than antibiotic treatment.

Equine uterine yeast infections may present with either yeast or hyphae. It is very uncommon to see both forms in one animal, since the individual uterine environment is usually only suitable for one type or the other.

95 a There is a monotonous population of small clear lymphocytes. There are two ovoid organisms with a wide mucoid capsule flanking a lymphocyte, and an internal structure at the top of the slide.
b Diagnosis: *Cryptococccus neoformans* infection associated with an atypical reactive T-cell hyperplasia. Differential diagnosis: *C. neoformans* associated with a small clear cell lymphoma.

96 a A multinucleated giant cell. Cells of this type in the smear contain from 10 to 20 or more nuclei. The cytoplasm is lightly basophilic and contains some green, granular material (source not identified). The nuclei vary from round to oval, but anisokaryosis or other markers of malignancy are not noted. The cells are considered to be Langerhans-type multinucleated giant cells.
b Granulomatous inflammation.
Note: In some cases with bizarre 'reactive' cells it may be difficult to differentiate a granulomatous inflammatory response from malignancy. In this case the uniformity of the nuclei and absence of features associated with malignancy supported an inflammatory reaction over neoplasia. In this case the green granular material (not pictured) was not specifically identified and special stains were not pursued. Granulomatous inflammation often arises when an underlying insult, organism or material cannot be resolved, and surgical removal may be required to achieve resolution. Knowledge of the type of inflammation and its significance is helpful in determining likely aetiologies and in planning the management and treatment of the case, and in client education.

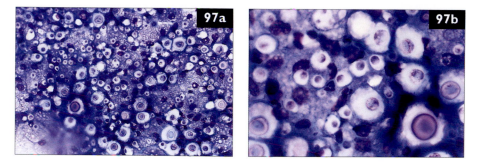

97 A 12-year-old cat presented with a subcutaneous, irregular, fluctuating swelling of the right side of the neck and right forelimb. Direct smears of the fluid collected from the lesion were stained for cytological examination (**97a, b**) (Wright–Giemsa, ×40 and ×100 oil, respectively).
a Identify the cell populations present, and describe the other features in this field.
b Classify the inflammatory response present. Does this provide any help with regard to the origin of the structures present in this field?
c What is your provisional diagnosis, and how might this be confirmed?

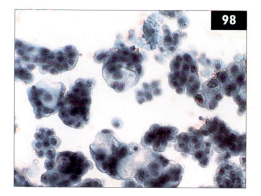

98 A 17-year-old Quarter Horse broodmare presented with unilateral mammary gland enlargement. The swollen gland was firm and slightly painful. An FNA was collected from the gland.
a Describe the cells and features seen in this smear (**98**) (Papanicolaou, ×100 oil).
b What is your interpretation of this aspirate?

97 a Highly vacuolated macrophages and neutrophils are present. The latter are seen more readily at the higher magnification. Note the round to oval structures with blue/purple central region, a clear halo and very variable size.
b There is evidence of a pyogranulomatous inflammatory response, which may be associated with fungal infection, mycobacterial infection, foreign body, panniculitis or protozoal infection. The structures present are consistent with fungal infection due to *Cryptococcus neoformans*.
c The presence of a pyogranulomatous response with variably sized organisms with a clear halo is consistent with a fungal infection. The morphology of the yeast forms is consistent with *C. neoformans*. Culture of material from the lesion produced a profuse growth of *C. neoformans*. Cryptococcosis can produce subcutaneous swellings, although it is more commonly associated with respiratory tract or neurological disease. The cellular response associated with infection is variable and, as in this case, the number of organisms may appear greater than the number of inflammatory cells. Cryptococcosis more commonly affects cats than dogs. The prognosis for feline cryptococcosis appears to have been improved by the use of fluconazole, but the owner of this cat requested euthanasia.

98 a There are a few erythrocytes and many cohesive papillary groups and rafts of cells. Some acinar configurations, with cells arranged around a clear space that is likely to be a lumen, are apparent. These cells have oval nuclei, usually with single small but distinct nucleoli. The cytoplasm is scant to moderate and varies from homogeneous to vacuolated. Some cells contain a single large cytoplasmic vacuole, while others contain multiple small vacuoles.
b The cytological features are consistent with mammary adenocarcinoma. This is an uncommon condition in the mare. Often, many neutrophils are present (not seen in this case) because there is concurrent mastitis; therefore, it may be difficult to diagnose in cases with overwhelming inflammation and few cells with features of malignancy. In this case a large number of malignant cells were obtained.

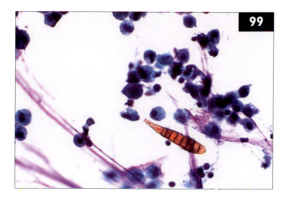

99 A five-year-old Thoroughbred-cross gelding presented for a tracheal washing. No history was included regarding the reason for obtaining the washing. A smear was made.
a What is the elongated, brown, segmented structure in the lower right/central portion of the smear (99) (Papanicolaou, ×100 oil)?
b What is the significance of this finding?

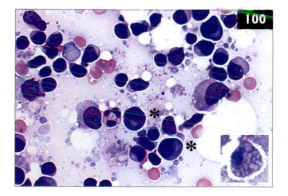

100 An FNA is collected from a prescapular lymph node of a six-year-old Terrier.
a Which interpretation best describes this smear (100) (Wright–Giemsa, ×50 oil): (a) normal; (b) reactive/hyperplastic; (c) metastatic tumour; or (d) multiple myeloma?
b What are Mott cells (insert in the right lower corner of the photomicrograph) and tingible body macrophages?
c List the differentials for reactive/hyperplastic lymph nodes.

99 a A fungal spore of the genus *Alternaria*.

b When present in small numbers these are considered to be an insignificant finding and should not be interpreted as evidence of fungal infection. When present in moderate to large numbers they may indicate an increased environmental load and/or decreased pulmonary clearance of environmental spores. Correlation with the spore and pollen count, evaluation to determine if mouldy hay may be present and consideration of environmental factors and other evidence of pulmonary disease may be needed to determine their significance when present in moderate to large numbers. Often they are accompanied by other types of spores and pigmented fungal hyphal fragments.

100 a (b) No clear line of separation exists between hyperplastic lymph nodes and 'normal' lymph nodes. Hyperplastic nodes are enlarged on clinical palpation and aspirates are usually highly cellular. In hyperplastic lymph nodes, small lymphocytes predominate and medium and large lymphocytes may be increased to contribute up to 15% of the lymphocyte population. Reactive lymph nodes are hyperplastic and have increased numbers of plasma cells (marked *) forming up to 5–10% of cells in some smears. Occasional Mott cells may be observed. Tingible body macrophages can represent >2% of the total nucleated cell population.

b Mott cells are plasma cells with basophilic cytoplasm in vacuoles called Russell bodies. The nature of Russell bodies is debatable but some authors suggest that they represent accumulations of immunoglobulins (Ig) within vesicles derived from rough interplasmic reticulum. The proposed underlying mechanism is a defect (partial or complete) in secretion of Ig. Tingible body macrophages are macrophages that contain phagocytosed remnants of DNA/cell debris. Increased numbers are seen with increased apoptosis/ 'cytorrhexis'.

c Differential diagnoses should include ehrlichiosis, FIV/FeLV infection, Rocky Mountain spotted fever and Lyme's disease.

Note: Tick-borne diseases are important differential diagnoses when lymphoid hyperplasia is observed cytologically. Other conditions that commonly result in generalized lymphoid hyperplasia include diffuse skin disease, external parasitism, fungal disease and systemic infection/sepsis. Generalized or regional lymph node enlargement with a cytological interpretation of hyperplasia may occur with tumour or localized irritation or injury. Idiopathic enlargement of lymph nodes may occur, and lymph node enlargement in young animals may occur as new antigens are encountered. In the absence of a specific cause for lymphoid stimulation recognizable in cytological preparations, continued investigation for an underlying cause is recommended.

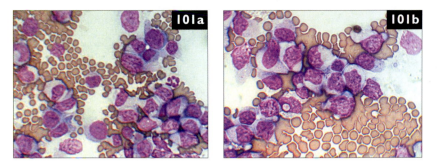

101 A 12-year-old neutered male Golden Retriever presented with generalized lymphadenopathy. An aspirate was collected from the prescapular lymph node.
a Describe what you see in these two smears (**101a, b**) (Wright–Giemsa, ×50 oil and ×100 oil, respectively).
b What is your interpretation?
c What cell type of origin is suspected based on the cellular morphology?
d What is the significance of this cell type of origin?

102 Pleural fluid is obtained from an eight-year-old cat with recent development of dyspnoea and pleural effusion. Analysis of the fluid revealed: TP = 52.2 g/l; albumin = 27.5 g/l;

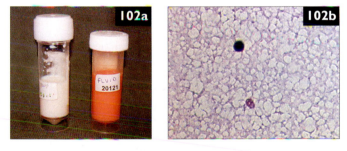

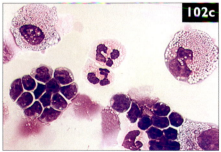

globulin = 24.7 g/l; albumin:globulin ratio = 1:1; SG = 1.040; WBCs = 54.96×10^9/l; RBCs = 0.28×10^{12}/l.
a Classify the pleural fluid.
b Based on the macroscopic (**102a**) and microscopic (**102b, c**) (Wright–Giemsa, ×50 oil and ×100 oil, respectively) appearance of the pleural fluid, which further laboratory tests would you like to request?
c Given the results of the tests requested above, how would you now reclassify this fluid?
d List the most common causes of chylous effusions in cats.

101 a The smears are of high cellularity. They contain a moderate number to many erythrocytes and many nucleated cells. The nucleated cells are discrete and have oval, angular, multiple indentations or slightly indented nuclei with clumped chromatin. Indistinct nucleoli are visible in some cells. The cytoplasm is moderate and palely to moderately basophilic. It does not have a darker rim or evidence of a perinuclear clear zone ('Golgi zone').
b These cytological findings are consistent with lymphoma.
c The features are consistent with T-cell origin. The angular and irregular nuclei, moderate cytoplasm without darker rim and area of perinuclear clearing are consistent with T-cell origin. The medium-sized lymphoid cells (nuclei approximately 2–3 times the diameter of the erythrocytes) and indistinct nucleoli suggest lymphoblastic subtype.
d In general, lymphomas of T-cell origin have a less favourable response to treatment than those of B-cell origin. Lymphoblastic T-cell lymphoma often presents with a mediastinal mass and paraneoplastic hypercalcaemia. Evaluation for these possibilities is indicated.

102 a An exudate. The TP is >30g/l and the NCC is >5×10^9/l.
b Fluid cholesterol and triglyceride concentrations.
c Chylous exudate. This interpretation is based on a fluid chylous:triglyceride ratio of <1 and a total triglyceride concentration of >1.13 mmol/l.
d Chylous effusions form when there is a physical (tumour, inflammation in mediastinum) or functional (cardiovascular disease) obstruction of lymphatics, resulting in increased pressure (lymphangiectasia) and, less commonly, rupture (trauma). In cats, cardiomyopathy is the most common cause.
Note: Identification of chylous fluid in a body cavity is consistent with lymph stasis. The body fluid analysis may reflect a modified transudate or exudate. The macroscopic milky appearance and presence of chylomicrons and lipid droplets cytologically may vary, depending on metabolic status and how recently a fatty meal has been consumed.

Sometimes, a fluid will have a similar appearance and be 'pseudochylous'. This is rare, but is associated with a higher cholesterol content than serum and may reflect increased cell turnover and breakdown of cell membrane lipids. It is usually the result of chronic irritation (pleuritis or peritonitis). Chylous effusions contain higher triglyceride levels compared with serum, which has a fluid:serum triglyceride ratio usually >3:1.

A variety of conditions and disease processes may result in chylous effusions, as noted above. In addition to cardiac insufficiency, the presence of a mass (abscess, haematoma, granuloma or tumour) interfering with vascular/lymphatic return and rupture of the thoracic duct, chylous effusions have been reported with diaphragmatic hernia, lung torsion, chronic coughing, chronic vomiting, steatitis, biliary cirrhosis, congenital lymphatic abnormalities, lymphangiectasia and as an idiopathic condition.

103 A six-year-old Bassett Hound presented for yearly examination and the owner mentioned the presence of a round firm nodule located on the right flank. The mass was 2.6 cm at its greatest dimension and firm on palpation. An FNA was collected and a smear made (**103**) (Wright–Giemsa, ×100 oil).

a Describe the cells present, and list the differentials.

b Would you consider this likely to be a malignant or a benign condition?

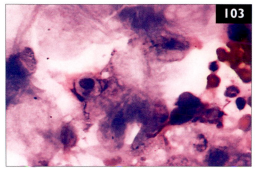

104 A four-year-old neutered female Siamese cat presents with a mass on its upper eyelid. A smear is made from an aspirate from the mass.

a Describe the cells seen in the smear (**104**) (Wright–Giemsa, ×100 oil).

b What is your interpretation?

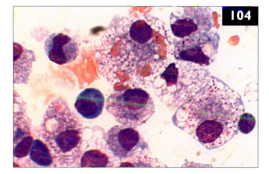

105 An aspirate is obtained from a fluctuant swelling on the head of a 15-week-old Mastiff puppy that had been bitten by a larger dog several days ago.

a What are these cells (**105**) (Diff-Quik, ×100 oil)?

b Can you characterize the type of inflammation?

c What are the organisms indicated by the arrows?

d Are they significant or artefactual?

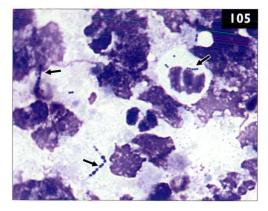

103 a The principal cell type is a keratinized squamous epithelial cell, and some of these cells retain small dense nuclei. There are also inflammatory cells present and these are mainly small lymphocytes. This is consistent with a benign keratinizing epithelial tumour or cyst. Surgical excision is always recommended as these may rupture and incite a foreign body response to the keratin.

b The presence of the majority of cells without nuclei or with small pyknotic nuclei supports a benign process.

Note: Keratinaceous material and squames (superficial anucleated squamous epithelial cells) may be seen in abundance, often in clumps, in aspirates from follicular or adnexal cysts or other types of keratinizing tumours. These cysts are nontumerous and may arise because of local irritation with blockage of adnexal or follicular ducts. In many cases the keratinaceous material and squames have a characteristic 'cheesy' appearance macroscopically. Sometimes, benign tumours of hair follicles or of squamous epithelial origin may contain cysts with similar contents.

104 a There are a few erythrocytes and plasma cells, with many large cells with vacuolated cytoplasm that resemble 'histiocytic' cells. They have oval nuclei, often with clumped chromatin. A single nucleolus is visible in some cells. Many of these cells contain a few to a moderate number of metachromatic cytoplasmic granules.

b The cytological features are consistent with aspiration from a mast cell tumour. The 'histiocytic' variety of mast cell tumour has been reported in cats and is more common in Siamese cats than in other breeds. It is important not to miss the metachromatic granules in these large, foamy cells. They must not be confused with macrophages; this would suggest chronic or granulomatous inflammation.

105 a The intact cells are neutrophils. Some of the smudged cells can also be recognized as neutrophils.

b Septic suppurative inflammation (an abscess).

c The short chains of cocci seen are probably *Streptococcus* species. Organisms are present extracellularly and within cells.

d Seeing bacteria inside neutrophils is probably significant. The presence of intracellular organisms is needed to confirm a septic condition.

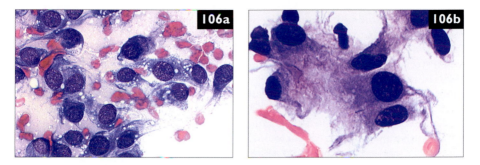

106 A seven-year-old female Springer Spaniel presented with a nodular intradermal/subcutaneous mass, approximately 10 cm in diameter, on the lateral surface of its elbow. An FNA was collected and smears made (**106a, b**) (Wright–Giemsa, ×50 oil and ×100 oil, respectively).

a Describe the cytological findings, and supply an interpretation.

b What is the most likely differential given the signalment, description of the mass and the cytological findings?

c Histology must be used to confirm the category of spindle/mesenchymal cell tumour. Why then is prior cytology useful?

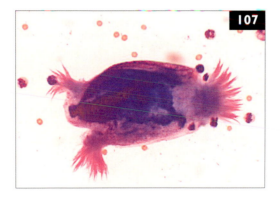

107 A seven-year-old Thoroughbred-cross gelding presented with a history of weight loss. A smear was made from the sediment from an abdominal fluid specimen.

a What is the structure shown (**107**) (Wright–Giemsa, ×50 oil)?

b What is the significance of this finding?

c What comments do you have regarding this finding?

106 a There are moderate numbers of mildly pleomorphic spindle shaped cells, loosely arranged with some features suggestive of a whirling pattern. Individual cells have a moderate nuclear:cytoplasmic ratio, single oval nuclei that are approximately two RBCs in diameter, coarsely stippled chromatin and a single medium sized nucleolus. They have moderate amounts of wispy basophilic, sometimes finely vacuolated, cytoplasm forming swirling tails.

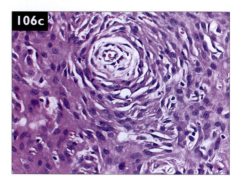

b Spindle/mesenchymal cell tumour.

c Haemangiopericytoma was confirmed on histology (**106c**) (H&E, ×50 oil). Haemangiopericytoma is a tumour that arises from pericytes (still inconclusive, could also be of neural origin). A multilobular nonencapsulated subcutaneous or dermal mass is identified histologically. Spindle/polygonal cells form whirls around capillary-sized lumens and are also arranged in short interlacing bundles and palisades. At low magnification, a characteristic 'finger print' pattern may be observed.

Information obtained on cytology can be helpful in the case management (i.e. appropriate perioperative planning [tend to bleed excessively] and aggressive surgical resection). Because most mesenchymal/spindle cell tumours tend to be infiltrative rather than metastatic, and particularly since local recurrence post surgical removal often has increasing invasiveness (one-fourth to one half of neoplasms recur four months to four years after surgical excision), knowledge of the potential biological behaviour is useful.

107 a A ciliated protozoan organism. Note the cilia at each orifice and the oesophagus and visible internal structure.

b This is likely to be the result of faecal contamination.

c The organism is probably present due to poor preparation of the paracentesis site or contamination of the tube with faecal material or faecally contaminated water. The possibility of aspiration of gastrointestinal content is considered unlikely, since there are not numerous bacteria (usually seen with gastrointestinal content aspiration) in the background. A repeat collection should be considered, with attention to hygiene, collection site preparation and specimen handling to prevent contamination.

108 A one-year-old female Pit Bulldog was presented with a history of anorexia, chronic vomiting and diarrhoea of three months' duration. Physical examination revealed mild icterus. Abdominal radiographs showed severe hepatomegaly and splenomegaly. Abnormal CBC findings included a moderate anaemia (PCV = 0.26 l/l). Abnormal biochemistry findings were: AST = 73 U/l (ref. = 14–38 U/l); ALT = 190 U/l (ref. = 10–71 U/l);

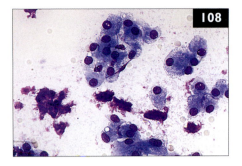

ALP = 2,047 U/l (ref. = 4–110 U/l); bilirubin = 29 µmol/l (ref. = 0–6.8 µmol/l). A smear was made from an FNA of the liver (108) (Wright–Giemsa, ×25).

a Describe the smear, and interpret your cytological findings.

b What stain procedure would help you confirm a diagnosis?

c Discuss the condition diagnosed.

109 A 19-year-old Clydesdale-cross gelding presented with a history of weight loss, partial anorexia and mild recurrent colic. An abdominal fluid sample was collected and analysis revealed: NCC = 15 × 10^9/l; TP = 40 g/l.

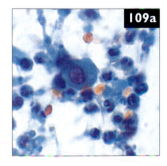

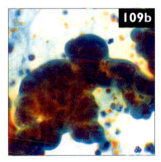

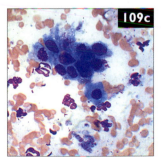

a Describe the features seen in these photomicrographs of the fluid (109a, b [Papanicolaou, ×50 oil and ×100 oil, respectively] and 109c [Wright–Giemsa, ×50 oil]).

b What is your interpretation of this specimen?

c What is the prognosis for this condition?

108 a The smear contains many hepatocytes with mild atypical features including anisocytosis, anisokaryosis and binucleation. Abundant homogeneous, pink extracellular material is noted in the centre of these hepatocyte clusters. The cytological interpretation is hepatic amyloidosis with presence of reactive hepatocytes.
b Congo Red specifically stains for amyloid. The eosinophilic material stained positive with Congo Red and was bright apple green when exposed to polarizing light.
c Amyloidosis is a disease characterized by the extracellular deposition of protein fibrils that have a specific configuration called the beta-pleated sheet. This configuration leads to the staining properties and insolubility of amyloid. Amyloid can be deposited in any organ. Organ malfunction develops as normal tissue is encroached upon by amyloid deposition. There are systemic and localized forms of amyloidosis. Localized amyloidosis is uncommon in dogs and cats. There are two systemic forms of amyloid; primary and secondary. Primary amyloid is derived from light chains of immunoglobulins in dogs and cats with plasma cell tumours. Secondary amyloidosis is also called reactive amyloidosis and occurs in patients that have a chronic infectious, inflammatory or neoplastic process. Serum amyloid A (SAA) protein is a precursor of reactive amyloid and is increased 100–1,000 times over normal in active inflammation. It is also possible that patients who develop reactive amyloid have impaired ability to degrade SAA. The dog in this case likely has reactive amyloidosis. In this case, once the disease was diagnosed, the owner declined any further investigation.

109 a The photomicrographs show a background with many erythrocytes. There are a moderate number to many nucleated cells. These include a moderate number of neutrophils and a few macrophages, with an additional population of cells that occur singly and in cohesive groups. These cells have features of malignancy. They have oval nuclei with clumped, dense chromatin and usually have a single, prominent nucleolus. The cytoplasm is moderate to moderately abundant and varies from ovoid to angular or slightly elongated. The single cell shows distinct squamous differentiation with angular, crisply defined cytoplasm.
b The cytological features are consistent with gastric squamous cell carcinoma.
c The prognosis for gastric squamous cell carcinoma is poor. Its presence in abdominal fluid indicates that there has been rupture of the stomach wall or rupture of lymphatics containing malignant cells. These are the avenues of access into the abdominal fluid.

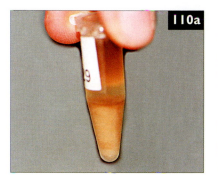
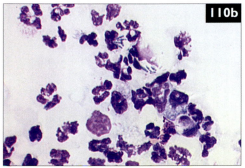

110 Abdominocentesis was performed on a cat with an inflammatory leukogram and a toxic left shift. Biochemistry revealed moderately increased ALP and ALT and mild azotaemia.

a Interpret the fluid specimen (110a) using the laboratory data and photomicrograph (110b) (Wright–Giemsa, ×100 oil). Fluid analysis: TP = 33.9 g/l; albumin = 14.1 g/l; globulin = 19.8 g/l; albumin:globulin ratio = 0.7; SG = 1.028; WBCs = 150.9×10^9/l; RBCs = 0.04×10^{12}/l.

b In view of the fact that the sample contained a pleomorphic bacterial population, including rods, cocci and filaments, select two further laboratory tests that you would like to run or be sent to a referral laboratory.

c What are the most common bacteria isolated from pyothorax and septic peritonitis?

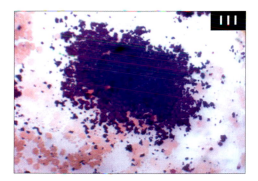

111 An ultrasound-guided liver aspirate is collected from an eight-year-old entire female Poodle. A smear is made from the aspirate.

a What is the material illustrated (111) (Wright–Giemsa, ×100 oil)?

b What is the significance of this finding?

c What comments do you have regarding this finding?

110 a Marked septic suppurative peritonitis. The bacteria have been phagocytosed and are therefore significant. Free bacteria may be contaminants.

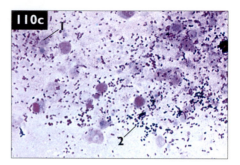

b (1) Gram's stain. These are gram-positive bacteria. Gram-negative (1) and gram-positive (2) bacteria, from two different lesions/patients, are shown in **KG15c** (Gram's, ×100 oil). Gram's staining allows the clinician to implement suitable interim antibiotics as part of a good therapeutic protocol. (2) Bacterial culture for both aerobes and anaerobes. A pleomorphic gram-positive bacterial population should alert the clinician to the possibility of *Actinomyces* or *Nocardia* infection.

c Dogs: *Escherichia coli*, *Pasteurella* species, *Actinomyces* species. Cats: aerobes: *Pasteurella* species, *Actinomyces* species, *Escherichia coli*; anaerobes: *Bacteroides* species, *Peptostreptococcus anaerobius*, *Fusobacterium* species.

Note: In some cases of pleural effusion due to *Actinomyces* or *Nocardia* infection, colonies of slender, beaded, filamentous or pleomorphic rods can be seen as soft, grey 'sulphur granules' with purulent exudate. These may be visible macroscopically, if large enough, as well as microscopically. Differentiation of *Nocardia* and *Actinomyces* is important, since different antibiotics are used for treatment. Standardization of Gram's and acid-fast (Ziehl–Neelsen) staining techniques is important in obtaining consistent and reliable results.

Nocardia organisms are found worldwide in soil. They stain Gram positive and are partially acid-fast. *Nocardia* species are often resistant to penicillin and cephalosporin but are usually susceptible to sulphonamides and potentiated sulphonamides.

Actinomyces organisms stain Gram positive but are acid-fast negative. They are usually susceptible to treatment with penicillin, clindamycin and cephalosporin, but are resistant to sulphonamides. They may appear to be inhibited by sulphonamides *in vitro*, but are not susceptible *in vivo*. Tetracyclines and erythromycin may also be used.

111 a Precipitate from ultrasound jelly.

b The precipitate is a contaminant from the skin preparation used for ultrasound evaluation.

c In some cases, ultrasound jelly precipitate may be so abundant that it obscures cellular and noncellular features. Other types of lubricants may have the same appearance. Careful collection and awareness of the possibility of contamination may help minimize the amount of material in ultrasound-guided collections.

112 An eight-year-old dog presented with clinical signs of pyrexia and a marked toxic leukogram with a degenerative left shift. Bronchoalveolar lavage was performed and smears made from the wash obtained.

a Identify the cells or structures labelled **1**, **2**, **3** and **4** in **112a** and **112b** (both Wright–Giemsa, ×50 oil), and state their significance in the context of a bronchoalveolar lavage.

b Interpret the pathological process seen in **112c** (Wright–Giemsa, ×100 oil).

c How do you know the bacteria present in this wash are likely to be significant?

d Are eosinophils more or less effective at phagocytosing and killing bacteria than neutrophils?

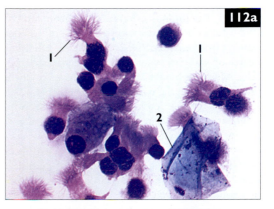

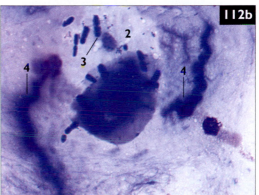

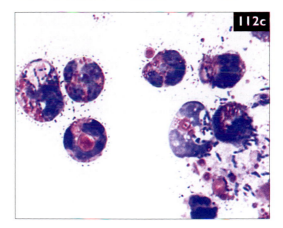

112 a 1 = columnar ciliated respiratory epithelial cells (confirms that the sample successfully obtained cells representative of the respiratory tract as far distally as the major airways [trachea, bronchi]; **2** = superficial squamous epithelial cell (indicates that there is a degree of oral contamination); **3** = the bacteria on the surface of the squamous epithelial cells, which are *Simonsiella* species; these are normal inhabitants of the oral pharynx and also indicate that the wash is contaminated; **4** = Curschmann's spirals (inspissated mucus).
b Marked, mixed, septic, predominantly eosinophilic respiratory tract inflammation.
c Bacteria are present within lysosomes, in the cytoplasm of eosinophils that have phagocytosed them.
d Less effective. Although eosinophils have receptors that allow them to phagocytize bacteria, they have a lower density of complement receptors than neutrophils and, despite high levels of peroxidase activity, oxidative responses and H_2O_2 than neutrophils involved in the killing process of bacteria, they lack several bactericidal substances (lactoferrin and phagocytin) and their cationic proteins have weak or no bactericidal or inflammatory properties.
Note: Curschmann's spirals are associated with conditions characterized by chronic and excessive production of mucus. They may occur in respiratory and reproductive cytology specimens and, in humans, have been reported in specimens from body cavity (pleural and peritoneal) fluids.

Superficial squamous epithelial cells, with or without bacteria, in respiratory cytology specimens are the result of oropharyngeal contamination in most cases. The amount of contamination may vary but, with experienced and careful collectors, is usually low.

Squamous metaplasia may occur in the respiratory system in response to chronic irritation. In this condition the columnar to cuboidal epithelium of the airways is replaced by stratified, flattened epithelium. It is usually a focal to focally extensive change. It is thought to represent an attempt at repair and protection from chronic irritation but may, in fact, lead to a nonfunctional and nonprotective epithelium that does not have normal secretion or mucociliary apparatus function. The development of squamous metaplasia is preceded by proliferation of reserve or basal cells, a change that may be visible as increased thickness and numbers of small, uniform, tightly cohesive cells with scant cytoplasm in tissue fragments. As these cells mature and differentiate, they resemble maturing squamous epithelium but are smaller and have a higher nuclear:cytoplasmic ratio. There may be an increase in granularity of chromatin and hyperchromasia and nucleoli may be present with increasing atypia and progression to dysplasia. In human studies, squamous metaplasia and dysplasia have been found to antedate the appearance of carcinoma of the lung. Severe dysplasia may mimic carcinoma or represent so-called bronchial intraepithelial neoplasia (BIN) that may, in some cases, progress to invasive cancer. These changes have not been studied in detail in dogs to see if the same potential biological behaviour and progression are present. However, squamous metaplasia has been recognized in respiratory cytology specimens from dogs and horses and is interpreted to represent a response to marked, chronic irritation.

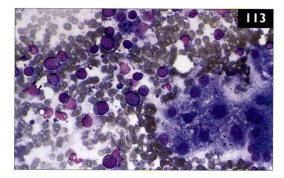

113 A six-year-old female Basset Hound presented for lethargy, decreased appetite and weight loss of two weeks' duration. Moderate hepatomegaly was detected on physical examination. A CBC revealed a slightly icteric serum, and a mild nonregenerative anaemia. On the biochemical profile, the liver enzymes ALT, AST and ALP were all moderately elevated. No other abnormalities were observed. An FNA was collected and a smear made (113) (Wright–Giemsa, ×25).
a Describe the cytological findings, and state your cytological interpretation.
b How is this condition cytologically different from the cat presented in case 41?

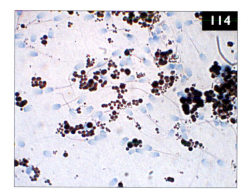

114 An eight-year-old entire male Border Terrier presented with a history of blood in the urine. An enlarged, irregularly shaped prostate gland was felt on palpation and a prostatic washing was collected.
a Describe the findings in this cytological preparation from the washing (114) (Wright–Giemsa, ×100 oil).
b What is the significance of these findings?
c What other recommendations might you have?

113 a The smear contains hepatocytes with indistinct cytoplasmic vacuolation and peripheral cytoplasmic clearing consistent with glycogen. Many lymphoblasts are infiltrated around the hepatocytes and are individually arranged with scant to moderate amounts of deeply basophilic cytoplasm. The nuclei are round to polygonal and usually two or more times the size of erythrocytes. The chromatin is typically diffuse and nucleoli are often seen. Low numbers of small, well-differentiated lymphocytes (about the same size as an RBC) are also noted. The cytological interpretation is hepatic lymphoma with vacuolar degeneration and mild cholestasis.
b Lymphocytic/plasmacytic hepatitis and cholangiohepatitis are characterized by a predominance of lymphocytes and plasma cells. Inflammation of this kind is more common in cats than in dogs. It is difficult to distinguish lymphocytic/plasmacytic inflammation from a well-differentiated lymphoma in cats. However, unlike the cat, in dogs, hepatic lymphoma most often involves an immature cell type (lymphoblast). In these cases the cytological diagnosis can be made with confidence.

114 a There is a moderate number of erythrocytes, in clumps, and many spermatozoa in the background. The spermatozoa have pale blue heads and pale grey tails, some of which are curled or have been detached. No neutrophils or infectious agents are visible.
b The spermatozoa are an incidental finding in a prostatic washing since there is usually ejaculation when the reproductive/urinary system is massaged prior to collection of a prostatic washing. The erythrocytes confirm the presence of blood, but no inflammation is seen.

No transitional epithelial cells are seen in this smear. They are often present in prostatic washings. In this case they were represented in other fields and did not have features consistent with malignancy. Sometimes, transitional cell carcinoma will occur in the prostatic urethra and grow or expand into the prostate gland. Therefore, evaluation of a prostatic washing is valuable because transitional epithelial cells from the prostatic urethra are usually represented.
c Since no columnar epithelial cells consistent with prostatic gland origin are seen, this precludes evaluation for features of hyperplasia or malignancy. If additional evaluation of the prostate gland is desired, ultrasound-guided fine needle aspiration of the prostate gland is recommended. This technique has a high probability of obtaining a representative specimen since it samples from the prostate gland directly. Ultrasound-guided FNAs of the prostate gland have replaced prostatic washings as the preferred specimen of choice for evaluation of suspected prostatic abnormalities and, since ultrasound is widely available, they are frequently submitted to the laboratory.

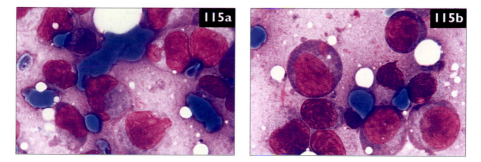

115 An FNA is collected from a canine cutaneous nodule.
a Describe the cells shown in these smears (115a, b) (May–Grünwald–Giemsa, ×100 oil).
b What is your diagnosis, and what are the differential diagnoses?

116 An eight-month-old castrated male Staffordshire Terrier-cross presented with patchy alopecia and erythema on its limbs and head.
a What is the organism shown (116) (1, egg; 2, nymph; 3, adult) (unstained skin scrape in mineral oil, ×10)?
b Why is it important to see multiple life stages?

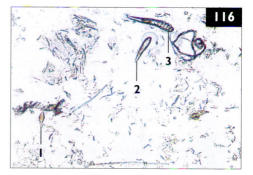

117 A five-year-old entire female German Shepherd Dog-cross presents with a history of chronic mucopurulent nasal discharge for six months. A smear is made from a nasal washing.
a Describe the features shown (117) (Wright–Giemsa, ×100 oil).
b What is your interpretation of these findings?
c What additional tests might be recommended?

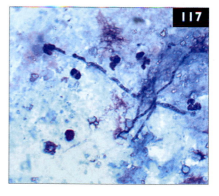

117

115 a Highly pleomorphic cells with nuclear lobations and deep indentations are evident in **115a**. The chromatin structure varies from delicate to moderately coarse. The nucleoli are poorly visible. The cytoplasm varies from pale to lightly basophilic. A clearly recognizable but atypical plasma cell is visible in the upper left corner. In **115b** the cells appear round and large with an extended deeply basophilic cytoplasm and a pale juxtanuclear area. The chromatin is more clumped in the smaller cell in the centre of the field.
b Diagnosis: malignant grade III plasmacytoma (cIg+). Differential diagnosis: mycosis fungoides would be a consideration based on the features seen in **115a**, but the plasmacytic differentiation is obvious in **115b** and would rule out mycosis fungoides, a tumour of T-cell origin.

116 a *Demodex canis*, the causative agent of so-called 'red mange' (demodicosis).
b It is important to see multiple life stages to confirm active proliferation consistent with infection. This follicular mite can also sometimes be found in skin scrapings of asymptomatic dogs. Multiple life stages as seen here indicate active proliferation. The adults have eight legs, the nymphs have six legs and the bodies are elongate.

117 a There is a mucoid background with a few neutrophils and erythrocytes. There is some refractile crystalline debris and several intertwined fungal hyphae. The hyphae are narrow (several microns in diameter) and irregularly septate. No branching is illustrated in these fragments, but in other fields the hyphae exhibited dichotomous branching.
b The features are consistent with active (neutrophilic) inflammation and the presence of fungal hyphae is suggestive of nasal aspergillosis.
c A fungal culture with evaluation of reproductive structures is needed for a definitive diagnosis of aspergillosis. Correlation with an *Aspergillus* antibody titre may be helpful in documenting exposure and an immune response to this organism. However, false-positive results may occur when there has been exposure but no current infection, and false-negative results may occur, particularly with early infection or infection in an immunocompromised animal that may not be capable of mounting an immune response. Correlation with the endoscopic appearance also may be helpful if white plaque-like lesions composed of fungal hyphae can be seen.

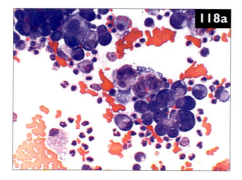

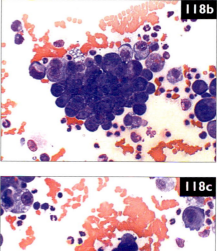

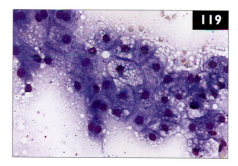

118 A nine-year-old spayed female Pug presented with a history of coughing, haemoptysis and dyspnoea. A bronchial washing was collected.
a Describe the cells shown in these three photomicrographs (**118a–c**) (all Wright–Giemsa, ×50 oil).
b What is your interpretation of these findings?
c What comment would you make about this condition?

119 A ten-year-old male mixed breed dog presented for surgical removal of the parathyroid gland following a diagnosis of parathyroid neoplasia. Biochemistry as part of presurgical screening revealed an elevated ALP (787 U/l). All other parameters were within normal limits. Thoracic radiographs were normal but abdominal ultrasound revealed several small nodules in the liver. A smear was made from an FNA of a nodule on the liver (**119**) (Wright–Giemsa, ×40).

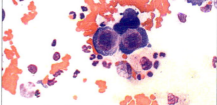

a Describe the smear, and interpret your cytological findings.
b Based on the ultrasound and cytological findings, what is the likely diagnosis?
c Discuss the aetiology for this condition.

118 a There are many erythrocytes and neutrophils, and many cells with features of malignancy. They occur singly and in cohesive groups, some with papillary configuration. These cells have oval nuclei with prominent nucleoli. The cytoplasm is moderate, oval and varies from homogeneous to finely vacuolated.

b The cytological features are consistent with pulmonary adenocarcinoma. The possibility of metastatic tumour that has broken through from the interstitium into the airway lumen cannot be completely ruled out, but the degree of cellularity is high and a primary pulmonary malignancy is most likely.

c Pulmonary adenocarcinoma often has metastases to other areas of the lung through blood vessels, lymphatics or airways. Bronchial lymph nodes are also often involved. Hypertrophic pulmonary osteopathy is a paraneoplastic syndrome that may accompany pulmonary adenocarcinoma. Excision is the treatment of choice if a single tumour mass is detected. Lobectomy is usually required to help achieve complete removal. If the disease is determined to be nonresectable at the time of surgery, there may be temporary palliation with incomplete excision. Chemotherapy may be used in these cases. The long-term prognosis for pulmonary adenocarcinoma is poor but the interval prior to death or euthanasia may be variable, extending up to 20 months in some reports.

119 a The smear contains several benign appearing hepatocytes, which have both distinct and indistinct cytoplasmic vacuolation suggestive of lipid and glycogen, respectively. Peripheral cytoplasmic clearing consistent with glycogen is also noted in several hepatocytes. Binucleation is also observed. Some distinct clear vacuoles consistent with lipid are seen in the background. The cytological interpretation is moderate hepatic vacuolar degeneration.

b A nodular lesion with a cytologically benign population of hepatocytes is the key to the diagnosis of nodular hepatic hyperplasia. Nodular hyperplasia is a focal proliferation of hepatocytes and is a common finding in old dogs. It is cytologically indistinguishable from hepatic adenoma. Hepatocytes often contain diffuse vacuolar degeneration, as noted in the figure, consistent with glycogen accumulation.

c The aetiology of spontaneously occurring hyperplastic nodules is unknown. However, nodular and hepatocytic hyperplasia can be experimentally induced by chemicals in a wide range of animal species. Specifically, nitrosamines and aflatoxin should be considered as potential causes of nodular hyperplasia, since these chemicals are frequently found in animal feeds, although the concentrations are generally low.

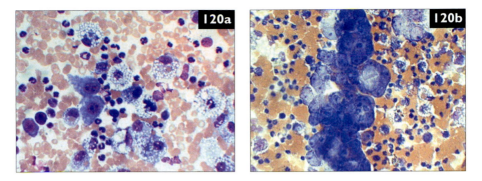

120 An eight-year-old entire female German Shepherd Dog-cross presents with a mammary mass. An aspirate is collected from the mass.
a Describe the features seen in these smears (**120a, b**) (both Wright–Giemsa, ×50 oil).
b What is your interpretation?
c What prognosis can you give?

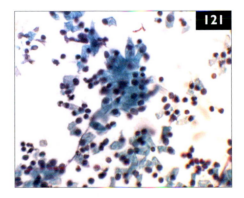

121 A three-year-old maiden mare arrives at a breeding farm in May. A uterine washing is collected to assess her reproductive status.
a Describe the features seen (**121**) (Papanicolaou, ×50 oil).
b What is your interpretation of these findings?
c Why is this important?

120 a There are bloody backgrounds with many erythrocytes and numerous neutrophils in **120a** and **120b**, as well as a moderate number of foamy macrophages in **120a**. The foamy macrophages may be associated with a cystic area with retained, phagocytosed secretion. In **120a** there are two discrete cells with ovoid to triangular, flocculant cytoplasm and oval nuclei containing coarsely clumped chromatin and one to several, distinct to prominent nucleoli. A large, cohesive group of cells with an acinar configuration is present in **120b**. These cells have features of malignancy, with distinct nucleoli, high nuclear:cytoplasmic ratio and moderate anisocytosis and anisokaryosis.
b The cytological features are consistent with mammary adenocarcinoma.
c Evaluation for metastases is recommended. If metastases are present, the prognosis is very poor. If metastases are not detected, there is reason for cautious optimism, since it is estimated that approximately 50% of mammary malignancies may be cured by complete removal. However, late-appearing metastases may occur, so continued monitoring is needed after removal in the event of the absence of current metastases.

Mammary malignancies may be obvious, as in this case; however, in some cases diagnosis may be difficult since the features of malignancy may be subtle and may not be present in all cells. Furthermore, caution in diagnosis is needed since inflammation may result in atypia that may mimic malignancy. If there is any atypia in a mammary mass, surgical removal with histological evaluation should be strongly considered in order to obtain a definitive diagnosis.

121 a Many columnar epithelial cells with oval, basal nuclei containing finely stippled chromatin can be seen. The cytoplasm is columnar and finely vacuolated. A few small lymphocytes are seen in the background. No neutrophils or infectious agents are visible.
b The cytological features are consistent with normal reproductive status and active cycling.
c It is important to know this since the cytology indicates that this mare is ready to breed and does not need any treatment prior to breeding. It is important to compare the results of uterine cytology with that of bacterial culture (often required by breeding farms upon entry). In this mare there was a scant growth of *Streptococcus* species obtained on culture, but the cytology indicates that this is likely to be a false-positive result since inflammation is not present. Correlation of the uterine cytology and culture is needed to determine if inflammation is present in the face of a positive culture. If so, treatment is indicated. If not, treatment is not indicated.

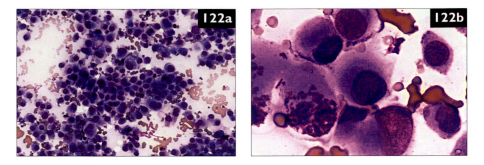

122 A three-year-old neutered male DSH cat presented with nodular masses on both the right forelimb (carpal region) and the left hindlimb (metatarsal region). Palpable nodules were also apparent at the point of the shoulder and under the jaw. The latter were considered to be lymph nodes. The cat was febrile with a temperature of 41°C (105.8°F) and it appeared to have lost weight since being examined six months previously. The cat had been inappetent and reluctant to play over the preceding week. Smears were made from aspirates taken from the nodules on the limb (122a, b) (Wright–Giemsa, ×10 and ×100 oil, respectively) and from the prescapular node. Describe the cell population, and outline the criteria for malignancy seen in the smears.

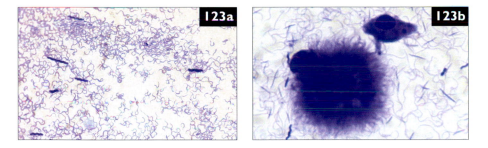

123 A ten-week-old Labrador Retriever puppy, just purchased from a pet store, presented with mucoid diarrhoea flecked with blood. The puppy was bright and alert and had a good appetite. On a direct saline mount of the stool, in addition to *Giardia* trophozoites there are thousands of motile, thin S-shaped rods, rapidly waving in the background (123a) (Diff-Quik, ×100 oil). There are a few structures (123b) (Diff-Quik, ×100 oil) that appear to be protozoa with hundreds of flagella.
a What are the bacteria?
b What are the 'protozoa'?

122 There is a discrete round cell population apparent, with many criteria for malignancy including bizarre mitoses, significant anisokaryosis, multiple nuclei and large nucleoli. There is no evidence of clustering of cells; hence the general term 'round cell' is applied. This population has too much cytoplasm to consider a lymphoid origin, so macrophages, osteoclasts, osteoblasts and chondroblasts should all be considered.

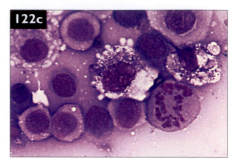

For comparison, a more typical view of a 'round cell tumour' is shown (122c) (Wright–Giemsa, ×100 oil). This is from a case of cutaneous histioyctosis in a six-year-old Golden Retriever. The variability is not as marked, although the condition is often associated with an aggressive growth pattern. The cells are 'round' in that they have no cytoplasmic attachments and have distinct cytoplasmic boundaries.

Note: The two examples of 'round cell' tumours shown in this case illustrate presentations of malignant 'round cells' in which it may be difficult to determine cell type origin based on the cytological features alone. A diagnosis of a poorly differentiated malignancy may be possible based on cytological features. Histological evaluation and/or special stains or other techniques may be needed to more accurately determine cell type of origin.

123 **a** Spirochaetes, recently renamed *Brachyspira* species. The previous genus name was *Serpulina*: two species are seen in the dog, *B. pilosicoli* and *B. canis*. Identification of the species requires culture and special tests.

b This is not a protozoan organism. *B. pilosicoli* can attach to epithelial cells by the apex of the bacterium. This is a sloughed epithelial cell showing hundreds of apically attached spirochaetes.

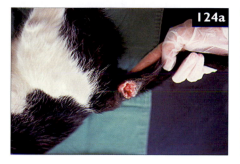

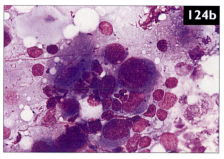

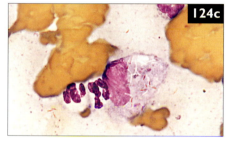

124 A five-year-old DSH cat has a number of firm nodular masses up to 3 cm in diameter in the subcutaneous tissue of the back, flanks and tail. Some are ulcerated (**124a**). An FNA is collected and smears made (**124b, c**) (Wright–Giemsa, ×50 oil and ×100 oil, respectively).
a What cells are present?
b What is your diagnosis?

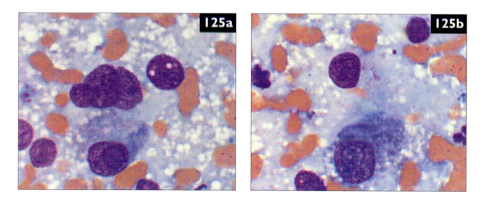

125 A seven-year-old neutered male Collie presented with an intra-abdominal mass. Smears were made from an aspirate from the mass.
a What is the large intranuclear structure in the cell in the lower central portion of these smears (**125a, b**) (both Wright–Giemsa stain, ×100 oil)?
b What is the significance of this structure?

124 a The smears are filled with reactive macrophages and lymphocytes, with some neutrophils and disrupted cells. The outline of nonstaining or lightly staining rod-shaped organisms can be seen in a macrophage in **124c**. A few extracellular organisms are present.

b Granulomatous inflammation. Subsequently, tissue from a surgical biopsy stained positively for mycobacterial organisms with Ziehl–Neelsen (acid-fast) stain, and a diagnosis of feline leprosy was made.

Note: Note the large nucleolus, high nuclear:cytoplasmic ratio and clumped chromatin in a macrophage in **124b**. In some cases it may be difficult to differentiate bizarre cells associated with granulomatous inflammation, epithelial injury, healing or repair from malignant cells. Consideration of the appearance of the other cells in the smear, the smear pattern (culmination of all cellular and noncellular material), the clinical appearance and other evaluations may be needed to help differentiate a bizarre reactive process from cancer in some cases.

If granulomatous inflammation is identified in a cat, mycobacterial infection should be part of the differential diagnosis. Careful scrutiny of smears and tissue sections may be needed to detect organisms, and additional investigation by Ziehl–Neelsen staining of aspirates and tissue sections should be pursued. Additional tests, such as PCR, may be needed to demonstrate infection when organisms are few.

125 a A cytoplasmic invagination producing an intranuclear cytoplasmic pseudoinclusion. These are sometimes called 'Orphan Annie eye' inclusions because they are reminiscent of the eyes drawn in the cartoon character Orphan Annie. They have been reported in specimens from humans, including thyroid carcinoma, meningioma, paraganglioma, pheochromocytoma and melanoma. Electron microscopic studies have shown these inclusions to include cytoplasmic organelles such as endoplasmic reticulum, Golgi apparatus and secretory granules.

b The significance of the intranuclear structure is that it should not be confused with a nucleolus. Features that help differentiate this structure from a nucleolus are the distinct surrounding membrane, the granular nature and the absence of darker staining that is usually seen with nucleoli.

126 A 13-year-old entire female Poodle-cross presented with a history of nasal discharge with sneezing. An area of bone lysis and soft tissue density was visible in the left nasal passage on radiography.

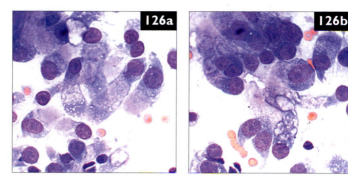

a Describe the cells illustrated (126a, b) (both Wright–Giemsa, ×100 oil).
b What is your interpretation?

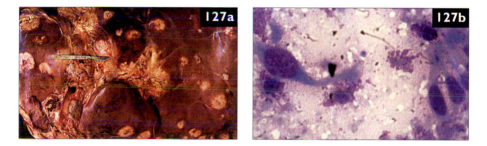

127 A thin, inappetent five-year-old Friesian cow was euthanased. On postmortem examination the liver was found to be studded with yellow masses (127a). An impression smear was made from one of these masses (127b) (Wright–Giemsa, ×50 oil).
a What cells are present?
b What is the cytological interpretation?

128 An FNA is collected from canine spleen.
a Describe the cells represented in this photomicrograph (128) (May–Grünwald–Giemsa, ×100 oil).
b What is your diagnosis, and what are the differential diagnoses?

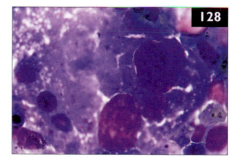

126 a The figures illustrate a specimen of high cellularity. The cells are tall columnar epithelial cells with oval, basal nuclei, within which a single distinct nucleolus is often visible. The nucleoli are round to slightly angular. The cytoplasm is columnar and varies from homogeneous to moderately vacuolated. There is moderate anisocytosis and anisokaryosis.

b These features are consistent with nasal adenocarcinoma. This appears to be a well-differentiated tumour. Nasal adenocarcinoma can vary from well-differentiated to poorly differentiated. Columnar cells with basal nuclear orientation are apparent in this case. It may be difficult to differentiate reactive columnar epithelial cells from well-differentiated adenocarcinoma in some cases. Consideration of the degree of cellularity, consistency of atypia, degree of atypia and other factors (clinical, radiography, etc.) may be needed to help determine if well-differentiated malignancy is present.

127 a The cells vary widely in size but are distinctly spindle shaped. They have tails of basophilic cytoplasm and oval nuclei with clumped chromatin. There is a lot of cell debris, suggesting cell fragility and necrosis.

b The presence of clusters of spindle-shaped cells alien to this position indicates a spindle cell tumour/sarcoma. A diagnosis of rhabdomyosarcoma was made on histopathological examination.

Note: Diagnosis of sarcoma, as mentioned in the discussion of other cases in this book, may be as specific a diagnosis as can be made based on routine cytological evaluation. In some cases of rhabdomyosarcoma there may be sufficient organization of intracytoplasmic filaments to demonstrate cross striations typical of skeletal muscle. This is usually only present in a few cells, if any. Immunohistochemical demonstration of myosin and desmin in the cells with malignant features is supportive of muscle origin, while demonstration of myoglobin is considered specific for muscle origin.

128 a There are two very large, atypical cells with a coarse chromatin and a poorly defined, extended and deeply basophilic cytoplasm. There are small lymphocytes in the background.

b Diagnosis: malignant histiocytosis (Rottweiler) (lysozyme +, NASDA +). Differential diagnoses: none in particular.

129 A ten-year-old spayed female Poodle presented with acute onset of paroxysmal sneezing. She was anaesthetized for nasal endoscopy and a nasal wash. Some of the saline retrieved was centrifuged and prepared for microscopic examination.

a What is the large cell, and what are the purple structures (**129a**) (Diff-Quik, ×100 oil)?

b Is it significant with regard to the dog's clinical signs?

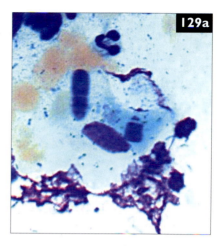

130 A three-year-old neutered female German Shepherd Dog-cross presented with a 3 cm × 6 cm mass located to the right of the sternum and extending up the chest wall. The dog was in good physical condition and was eating well. The owner had only just noticed the mass. An FNA was collected and smears made (**130a, b**) (Wright–Giemsa, ×50 and ×100 oil, respectively).

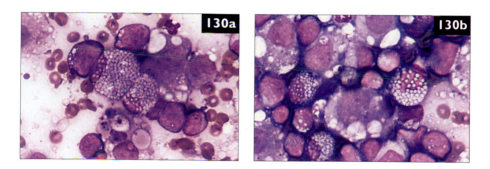

a Describe the cells present. What might they represent?

b Would you consider this to represent a benign process? If so, why?

129 a The large trapezoidal cell is a squamous epithelial cell and the purple structures that look like stacked coins are palisades (they divide side-to-side instead of forming chains) of a bacterium called *Simonsiella*.

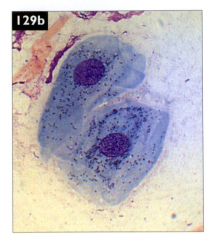

b No. It is a normal commensal of the oropharynx and is an often-seen contaminant in specimens from the oropharynx, nasal cavity or respiratory collections that pass through the oropharynx.

Note: *Simonsiella* species are usually noted because of their distinctive and large appearance. This photomicrograph (**129b**) (Wright–Giemsa, ×100 oil) shows some large squamous epithelial cells with numerous green to green-black small granules consistent with melanin. For inexperienced cytologists, these may be confusing and melanin granules may be mistakenly identified as bacteria.

130 a The cells are a mixture of round cells, which include macrophages (some of which have cytoplasmic vacuoles and material), small lymphoid cells and lymphoblasts, and plasma cells, which contain Russell bodies. RBCs are also present, which can be used to estimate the size of the other cells (6 μm diameter). The mixed cell population and the presence of plasma cells with Russell bodies suggest a granulomatous inflammatory reaction. The Russell bodies are thought to be collections of immunoglobulin.

Causes of granulomatous inflammatory reactions include infectious agents such as fungal elements, rickettsiae and parasites; noninfectious conditions such as ruptured keratin cysts, foreign body reactions, pancreatitis (nodular panniculitis) and immune-mediated conditions; and finally neoplastic conditions such as systemic or cutaneous histiocytosis.

b Yes. Although age does not completely rule out the possibility of neoplasia, the young age of the dog and the appearance of the granulomatous inflammation suggest that this is a benign process. There are no features that suggest malignancy.

Note: Sometimes an underlying cause or infectious agent will be apparent in cytological preparations, but other cases will only show a nonspecific pattern.

131 A two-year-old Schnauzer-cross presented for inappetence, severe bloody diarrhoea and weight loss. The temperature on admission was 39°C (102.2°F) and the animal appeared to have abdominal pain on palpation. Nonproductive vomiting was also present. A CBC revealed a modest neutrophilia with monocytosis and biochemistry showed marginally low TP and albumin without proteinuria or

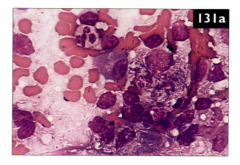

alteration in liver enzymes. The dog was treated with antibiotics and fluid therapy and, over the next few days, the diarrhoea diminished but the lymph nodes, both prescapular and mandibular, enlarged. Aspiration of a lymph node was performed and a smear made (**131a**) (Wright–Giemsa, ×100 oil).

a Describe the cells and features that are present.

b What special stain would you use to confirm a diagnosis?

132 A 15-week-old Malamute puppy, just acquired from a 'backyard breeder', presented with itching and dermatitis. Flea combing revealed this organism (**132**) (unstained smear in mineral oil, ×40).

a What is the organism?

b Do the cats in the household need to be treated now as well? What about any children in the household?

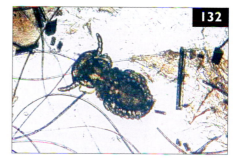

133 An aspirate is collected from a red, slightly raised, poorly defined lesion on the right upper lip of a two-year-old neutered male DSH cat.

a Describe the features illustrated (**133**) (Wright–Giemsa, ×50 oil).

b What is your interpretation of these findings?

c What differential diagnoses are you considering based on these findings?

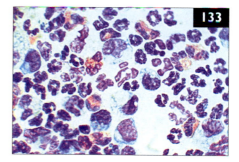

131 a There are a few neutrophils and many macrophages. The macrophages contain linear 'ghost' outlines seen with organisms that have a thick capsule with a high lipid content.

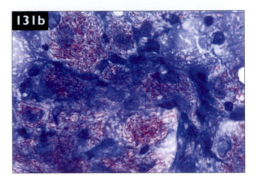

b An acid-fast (e.g. Ziehl–Neelsen) stain. An acid-fast stain superimposed on the Wright–Giemsa-stained smear (**131a**) is shown (**131b**). This is consistent with a *Mycobacterium* infection, and in this case the organisms were identified on culture as *M. avium-intracellulare* complex.

Note: Mycobacterial infections may vary greatly in the numbers of organisms that are present. PCR testing may be used to confirm suspected infections when organisms are too few to be demonstrated cytologically or histologically. Tuberculin skin tests are not consistently reliable in dogs, cats and horses.

Cats are resistant to infection with *M. tuberculosis*, but are susceptible to *M. bovis*, *M. avium* complex or *M. microti*. There are some other mycobacterial species that have also been isolated from cats. Contaminated milk has been implicated in causing gastrointestinal lesions and haematogenous dissemination to other organs. Some types of mycobacterial species are ubiquitous in soil and may contaminate skin or penetrating wounds.

132 a A chewing louse, consistent with *Trichodectes canis*.
b No, the cats and kids do not need to be treated. These lice are quite host-specific and cannot infest cats or humans.

133 a There are a moderate number to many neutrophils with a moderate number of eosinophils and macrophages. There are a few plasma cells in the lower left quadrant of the smear. No infectious agents are visible.
b The cytological features are consistent with pyogranulomatous and eosinophilic inflammation.
c The primary concern is feline eosinophilic granuloma complex. However, this type of inflammation in a cytological specimen may also occur with a reaction to a foreign body or a penetrating wound or with allergy.

134 An abdominal fluid specimen is collected at postmortem examination from an 11-year-old entire female DSH cat.
a Describe the cells illustrated (134) (Papanicolaou, ×100 oil).
b What is your interpretation?
c What is the significance of this finding?

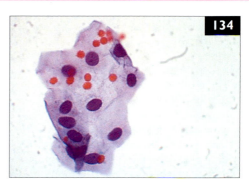

135 Uterine cytology was performed for routine assessment when a seven-year-old mare that had her third foal last year arrived at the stud farm prior to breeding.
a Describe what you see in these smears (135a, b) (both Papanicolaou stain, ×100 oil).
b What is your interpretation of these findings?
c Why is this good to know?

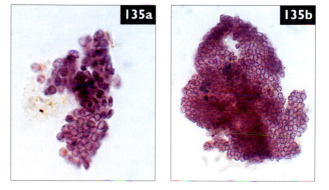

136 An FNA is collected from a canine lymph node.
a Describe the cells represented in this photomicrograph (136) (May–Grünwald–Giemsa, ×100 oil).
b What is your diagnosis, and what are the differential diagnoses?

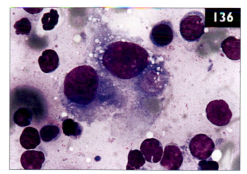

134 a There are a few erythrocytes and a group of delicate, flat epithelial cells that exhibit tight intercellular cohesion. They have central, oval nuclei with delicate chromatin. Nucleoli are absent, small or inconspicuous. The cytoplasm is moderate to abundant and pale blue-grey.

b These cells are consistent with mesothelial origin. The flat group may have been traumatically exfoliated. With increasing postmortem interval there may be spontaneous exfoliation of such groups, with hypoxia and autolysis. Sometimes, traumatically exfoliated groups of mesothelial cells with a 'flat' appearance of a raft of cells may occur with collection from a live animal, particularly in cows and horses where large-bore needles or teat cannulas may be used for collection, or in specimens collected at exploratory laparotomy. Mesothelial cells that have exfoliated into the abdominal fluid are usually 'rounded up' or occur in three-dimensional clusters, rather than as flat sheets.

c The presence of such a group of mesothelial cells in a postmortem collection is an insignificant finding. Other cell types and noncellular contents need to be considered. Careful interpretation of postmortem collections is recommended since there may be changes due to artefact or autolysis that may mimic pathological conditions.

135 a There are groups of epithelial cells with oval, hypochromatic 'bland' nuclei without granular chromatin or nucleoli. The cytoplasm is insubstantial and the boundaries are indistinct. The nuclei are often overlapping or very close together.

b These features are consistent with inactivity of winter anoestrus.

c This is good to know because it indicates that this mare is not ready to breed. The mare may need to be put under light or undergo hormone treatment, or it may be necessary to wait for her to come naturally into active reproductive physiological activity.

136 a There are two atypical spindle cells amongst a background of small lymphocytes. Note the large size, the nucleoli and the deeply basophilic and vacuolated cytoplasm.

b Diagnosis: metastatic lymphadenopathy from a poorly differentiated sarcoma. Differential diagnoses: metastatic lymphadenopathy from a spindle cell amelanotic melanoma; reactive fibroblasts in a fibrous lymph node.

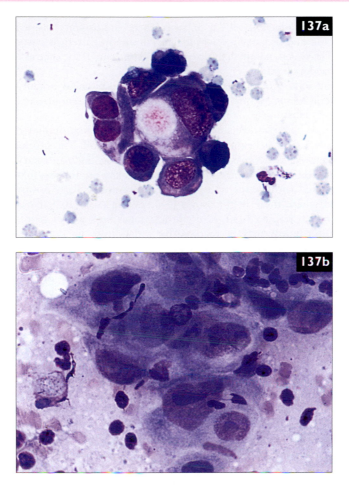

137 A ten-year-old crossbred bitch presented with haematuria that was nonresponsive to antibiotic therapy. A midstream, voided, urine sample was collected for initial analysis. Many epithelial cells were noted on examination of the urinary sediment, and a smear was prepared.
a Describe the cells identified (137a) (Wright–Giemsa, ×100 oil).
b What is your provisional diagnosis?
c What other tests may provide supportive evidence or definitive diagnosis?
d What prognosis is associated with this diagnosis?

137 a A cluster of adherent cells is present. There is anisokaryosis, a high nuclear: cytoplasmic ratio and prominent nucleoli. The chromatin pattern is particularly coarse in four cells. The round, pale staining area in the cytoplasm of the central cell is likely to reflect hydropic degeneration.

b The adherent nature of the cells is consistent with epithelial origin and there are sufficient criteria to suggest malignancy. Given the body system affected, transitional cell carcinoma is most likely.

c Double contrast radiographic studies or ultrasound examination may be useful, and in this case revealed a thickening of the dorsal bladder wall. The cytological features are highly suggestive of neoplasia, but in less convincing cases a urinary dipstick test may be employed. This latex agglutination test detects an antigen (bladder tumour antigen) associated with canine transitional cell carcinoma. False-positive test results may be noted where there is glucosuria (4+), pyuria (>30–40 leukocytes per high power field) or haematuria (>30–40 erythrocytes per high power field). Histological examination of a biopsy may be required for a definitive diagnosis. In this case the histological diagnosis was transitional cell carcinoma.

d Transitional cell carcinoma has a guarded to poor prognosis. It may be multifocal, with some sites not apparent macroscopically. There is potential for metastasis, often to regional lymph nodes of the abdomen and pelvis, or to the long bones or pelvic bones. Hypertrophic osteopathy may also occur. Some cases may respond to surgery if a single lesion is present, while others may show remission with piroxicam treatment.

Note: A photomicrograph (**137b** [Papanicolaou, ×100 oil], see page 135) from another dog with transitional cell carcinoma is included here for comparison. The smear contains small numbers of erythrocytes and many nucleated cells consistent with transitional epithelial origin, and it has features of malignancy. These cells show mild anisocytosis, with an increased nuclear:cytoplasmic ratio. The nuclei are large and oval, with prominent chromatin clumping and some uneven thickening of nuclear membranes. One or more distinct nucleoli are often present. The cytoplasm varies from scant to moderately abundant and is granular to finely vacuolated. A few binucleated cells are seen. The nuclear details may be more easily evaluated with haematoxylin staining (the nuclear stain used in the Papanicolaou stain) than with Romanowsky stains. The large cohesive group is the result of gentle traumatic exfoliation with a catheter in the area of a mass demonstrated radiographically. Individually exfoliated cells tend to 'round up' in the urine, while traumatically exfoliated groups more commonly appear as flat, cohesive groups of cells. This method of collection is beneficial in obtaining large numbers of cells for cytological evaluation. The urine specimen was immediately fixed by the addition of two drops of 10% buffered formalin per ml of urine specimen. The fixation helps preserve cells during transport to the laboratory. Papanicolaou staining is not routinely available in commercial laboratories in North America, but is available at several laboratories in the UK and continental Europe. The use of various stains and fixatives varies, depending on pathologists' preference, experience and training.

138 A three-year-old entire male Collie-cross presented with suspected biliary duct obstruction following surgery for removal of an intestinal foreign body. A gallbladder aspirate was collected.
a Describe the features shown in this smear (**138**) (Wright–Giemsa, ×100 oil).
b What is your interpretation of these findings?

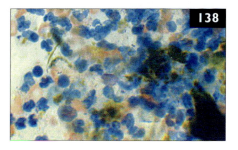

139 A four-year-old entire male Cocker Spaniel presented with a history of recurrent ear infections. A smear was prepared from a swab from the left ear.
a Describe the features illustrated (**139**) (Wright–Giemsa, ×100 oil).
b What is your cytological interpretation?
c What recommendations do you have regarding this condition?

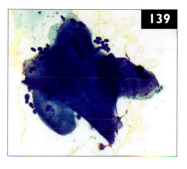

140 Pleural fluid is collected from a one-year-old cat with pleural effusion.
a Review the laboratory data and photomicrograph (**140**) (Wright–Giemsa, ×100 oil) and give an appropriate interpretation. Fluid analysis:
TP = 40.9 g/l; albumin = 23.2 g/l; globulin = 17.7 g/l; albumin:globulin ratio = 1.3; SG = 1.030; WBCs = 17.76 × 10^9/l; RBCs = 0.32 × 10^{12}/l.
b What are the sensitivity and specificity

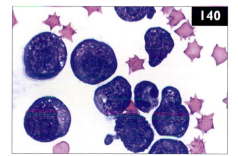

of cytological evaluation for the detection of malignant tumours in body cavity effusions of dogs and cats?
c Given the young age of this cat and the anatomical location of the lymphoma, what other laboratory data would you like to obtain that may affect the prognosis of this patient?
d Are FeLV-associated thymic mediastinal lymphomas in young cats B-cell or T-cell tumours?

138 a There are clumps of inspissated green pigment consistent with bile. There are a few erythrocytes and many poorly preserved and moderately degenerate neutrophils.

Bile aspirates are recognized by green colour macroscopically. Cytologically, normal bile often appears as granular blue to blue-grey or blue-green material. As it becomes inspissated or sludges with bile stasis or obstruction, clumps of green pigment and some bilirubin crystals become apparent.
b The features are consistent with marked, purulent inflammation with bile inspissation. The features are suggestive of septic cholecystitis. Some intracellular bacteria are found in other fields, confirming the presence of sepsis.

139 a There is a squame (anucleated squamous epithelial cell) in the centre of the picture. Associated with it are numerous, small 'footprint-shaped' yeast cells consistent with *Malassezia pachydermatis* infection.
b Fungal otitis.
c Specific antifungal treatment should be instigated. Attention to hygiene is needed, and excessive ceruminous and keratinaceous material should be minimized or eliminated, if possible, in order to help treat the infection and prevent possible recurrence or relapse of the condition following successful treatment.

140 a Lymphoma with secondary exudative effusion.
b Sensitivity (dog = 64%; cat = 61%); specificity (dog = 99%; cat = 100%). Therefore, the sensitivity is moderate but the specificity is good.
c The cat's FeLV status. 80% of cats with thymic mediastinal lymphomas are FeLV positive. Cats with FeLV negative status have a better prognosis. This is currently under review as there is contradiction between early and current literature. Some publications claim that the discrepancy is related to the decreasing incidence of FeLV-related lymphoma.
d T-cell tumours.
Note: The large discrete 'round cells' illustrated in this case are typical of malignant lymphoid cells. Based on the age, presence of a mediastinal mass and appearance of the cells, lymphoma is the correct interpretation. In some cases, malignant lymphoid cells may be difficult to differentiate from poorly differentiated malignant cells of mesenchymal or epithelial origin.

141 A 12-year-old Thoroughbred-cross broodmare presented with a history of repeated uterine infections. She displayed poor perineal confirmation, with a sunken anus. A uterine washing was collected to determine the mare's status prior to breeding.

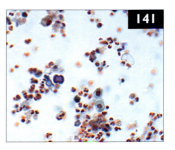

a What features are present in this smear (141) (Papanicolaou, ×50 oil)?

b What is your interpretation of these findings?

c What is the significance of these findings?

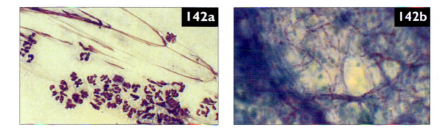

142 A seven-year-old neutered male Staffordshire Bull Terrier presented with a history of nasal discharge. White plaques were visible on retropalatal endoscopy. Smears were prepared from nasal swabs.

a Describe the features seen in the smears (142a, b) (both Wright–Giemsa, ×100 oil).

b What is your interpretation?

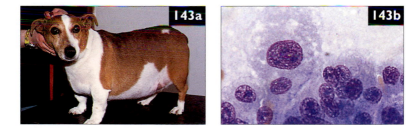

143 A neutered female crossbred terrier (143a) is dull and has abdominal enlargement. Hepatomegaly is noted on radiological examination. An FNA is collected from the liver and a smear made (143b) (Wright–Giemsa, ×100 oil).

a What cells are present?

b What is your diagnosis?

141 a There are many neutrophils with a few macrophages. In the centre left portion there are two noncellular structures – one stains purple and the other is green and appears to be composed of two segments or rounded portions that merge at their centres. Neither of these contains a nucleus.
b These two structures are urine crystals. These features and inflammation are associated with intrauterine urine pooling.
c This finding is significant since it indicates that surgical repair will likely be needed to prevent continued or periodic urine pooling and repeated infections. The poor perineal confirmation contributes to this condition. Urine is often present in the anterior vagina on speculum examination, but sometimes the primary diagnosis is made on the basis of cytological findings and no urine is apparent macroscopically.

142 a One smear (**142a**) contains a moderate number of neutrophils and a few macrophages. The other smear (**142b**) contains a large mat of fungal hyphae. The hyphae are narrow, septate and dichotomously branching.
b The cytological features are consistent with mycotic rhinitis with moderate, chronic and active inflammation. The morphology of the fungal elements is suggestive of aspergillosis. A definitive diagnosis will require staining with special preparations (Lactol Phenol Cotton Blue) and examination of reproductive structures. A positive aspergillosis titre would provide additional support for exposure to this organism, but a negative titre does not rule out the possibility of this condition. False-positive titres may occur since the presence of antibody only indicates prior exposure and does not confirm the presence of infection.

143 a The cells show marked anisocytosis and anisokaryosis. They have variably basophilic cytoplasm and some are multinucleated. Nuclear chromatin is clumped and large, sometimes multiple, nucleoli are seen. These are interpreted to represent malignant hepatocytes.
b Hepatic carcinoma.

144 An aspirate is collected from a cystic mass on the lumbar area of a six-year-old entire male Border Collie.
a Describe the cytological findings (144) (Wright–Giemsa, ×50 oil).
b What is the significance of these findings?
c What is your cytological interpretation, and what are your comments?

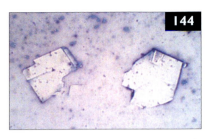

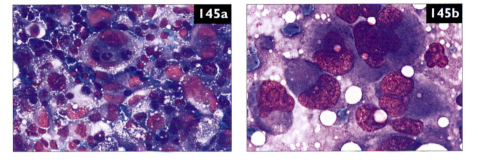

145 An FNA is collected from a pulmonary mass.
a Describe the cells in these smears (145a, b) (May–Grünwald–Giemsa, ×40 and ×100 oil, respectively).
b What is your diagnosis, and what are the differential diagnoses?

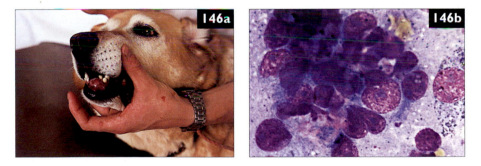

146 An aged Labrador has a firm painless mass on its gum (146a). An FNA is collected and a smear made (146b) (Wright–Giemsa, ×100 oil).
a What cells are present?
b What is your diagnosis?

144 a There is a slight protein background with several crystals that are flat, clear plates with 'notched corners'. These are consistent with cholesterol crystals.
b Cholesterol crystals may be seen in cysts with static secretion. They may be seen in areas with increased cell turnover and breakdown of lipid-containing cell membranes.
c Based on the cytological features, the interpretation would be consistent with origin from a secretory cyst. There is no current indication of inflammation or infection. Cells that would suggest a lining for, or origin for, a cyst are not seen. The possibility of adjacent tumour that is not represented in this collection cannot be ruled out, but many cysts with this cytological appearance are non-neoplastic in origin. They are not expected to resolve spontaneously; therefore, surgical removal with histological evaluation should be considered.

145 a A dense and highly atypical cell population is seen in **145a**. The cells have a great variation in size, with numerous giant cells, and they show an extreme nuclear pleomorphism. The cytoplasm appears extended, pale to highly basophilic and vacuolated. A very large cell in the upper centre shows intense leukophagia. At high magnification (**145b**) the round cell aspect, the reticular chromatin, the basophilia of the cytoplasm and the nuclear pleomorphism are obvious.
b Diagnosis: malignant histiocytosis (Bernese Mountain Dog). Differential diagnosis: none.

146 a There are a few RBCs but nearly all the nucleated cells are from a single population of pleomorphic cells. They are round to spindle shaped and there is anisocytosis and anisokaryosis. Cytoplasmic basophilia varies and there is chromatin clumping and some prominent nucleoli. A few cells (see cell at far right in **146b**) contain blue-green granules consistent with tyrosine-containing melanin precursors.
b A poorly differentiated melanoma.
Note: Poorly differentiated, amelanotic or poorly melanotic melanomas are 'great pretenders' and may have features that suggest epithelial and/or mesenchymal origin cytologically. As in this case, diligent searching may result in the identification of a few cells with small numbers of melanin granules or blue-green material consistent with melanin. In other cases, melanoma may be suspected but melanin not demonstrated.

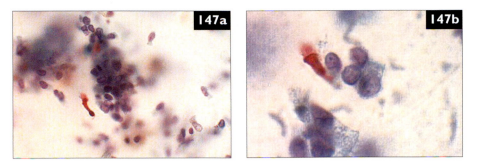

147 A five-year-old Quarter Horse broodmare that has not conceived during the current breeding season presents in September to determine whether treatment may be needed in preparation for breeding the following year. A uterine washing is collected.

a What features are present in these smears (**147a, b**) (Papanicolaou, ×50 oil and ×100 oil, respectively).

b What is your interpretation of these findings?

c What is the significance of these findings?

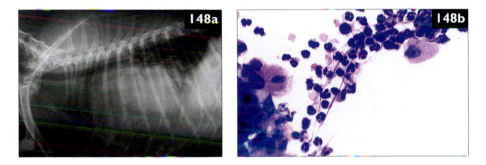

148 A lady runs a riding stable and her two-year-old entire male Jack Russell Terrier usually accompanies her on rides. The dog is presented because of exercise intolerance and mild respiratory distress.

a On auscultation, the dog's respiratory sounds are dull or absent in some lung fields. Review the chest radiograph (**148a**) and note any concerns.

b An FNA is collected from the thoracic cavity to help determine the cause of the respiratory distress. Describe your cytological findings and supply an interpretation (**148b**) (Wright–Giemsa, ×50 oil).

c Under what other circumstances might you aspirate a similar population of cells?

147 a There are low columnar to cuboidal epithelial cells that occur singly and in groups. The nuclei are relatively bland and chromatin stippling is not present. **147a** shows red to red-orange-staining (orangophilic) ciliated columnar epithelial cells with a basal, pyknotic cytoplasm. **147b** shows an orangophilic ciliated cytoplasmic tuft that has pinched off from the basal portion of the cell. No inflammatory cells or infectious agents are visible.

b The cytological features are consistent with fall transition.

c The significance of this finding is that this mare is past conceiving for the current year. The absence of inflammation suggests that treatment is not needed at this time. However, it does not rule out the possibility of increased susceptibility to infection following breeding. Re-evaluation after the onset of cyclic activity and prior to breeding is recommended.

148 a There is loss of the diaphragmatic line, loss of the cardiac silhouette and dorsal displacement of lung fields. There is no evidence of gas, nor was there evidence of barium on a follow-up barium free-flow study. It is unclear whether this is an abscess, haemorrhage or a hernia.

b There are moderate numbers of mildly degenerate neutrophils intermittently associated with low numbers of large polygonal shaped cells. The latter have a moderate nuclear:cytoplasmic ratio, a single round nucleus, indistinct nuclear features and moderate amounts of slightly granular eosinophilic cytoplasm. In some cells, particularly in the cluster to the left of the photomicrograph, moderate amounts of green/ black globular pigment are superimposed on the clusters and within the cytoplasm of polygonal cells. Interpretation: moderate suppurative pleuritis, possibly secondary to diaphragmatic hernia. The polygonal cells are hepatocytes and the black pigment is bile.

c When performing fine needle aspiration of the thoracic cavity, particularly when the needle is inserted in the caudal portion, and especially in cats, accidental aspiration of abdominal content can occur. This should not be confused with metastatic tumour.

Further investigation revealed that the dog had received a kick from one of the horses, likely resulting in the diaphragmatic hernia.

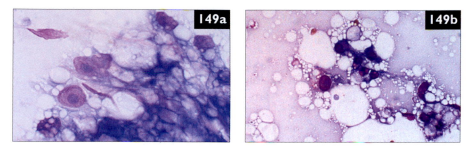

149 An aspirate is collected from a rapidly growing mass on the left thorax of a six-year-old entire female Boston Terrier.

a Describe the features seen in these two smears (149a, b) (Wright–Giemsa, ×50 oil and ×100 oil, respectively).

b What is your cytological interpretation?

c Are there any confirmatory tests that can/should be done?

d What is the expected biological behaviour?

150 A ten-month-old male Labrador Retriever presented with a lump on the back of its head. An FNA was collected from the mass.

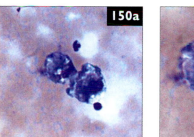
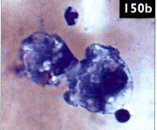

a Describe the features illustrated in these two photomicrographs (150a, b) (Wright–Giemsa, ×50 oil and ×100 oil, respectively).

b What is your interpretation?

c What comment would you make about this condition?

151 A six-year-old rescued Boxer was seen as a second opinion for chronic, lifelong generalized demodicosis. She was on daily ivermectin and had recovered some of her hair. A skin scrape was taken.

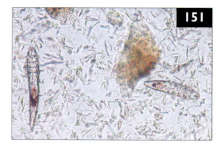

a Describe the organisms shown (151) (unstained smear in mineral oil, ×40).

b What is the significance of the difference in size?

145

149 a There are slight protein backgrounds with lipid droplets and individual cells and cells in groups that have features of malignancy. There are large, oval nuclei, often with a single, prominent nucleolus. The cytoplasm is moderate, elongated and often contains one or several crisply defined vacuoles.
b A sarcoma. The lipid vacuoles and vacuolated cytoplasm are highly suggestive of liposarcoma.
c Sudan III staining of an unfixed, air-dried smear would be able to confirm the presence of lipid. The Sudan III stains lipid red to pink.
d Evaluation for possible metastasis is recommended. Metasteses are not common. If none is observed, wide and deep surgical excision is the recommended treatment.

150 a There are very bloody backgrounds with many erythrocytes and a relatively low density of nucleated cells. There are a few neutrophils, lymphocytes and macrophages, and a few erythrophages. No infectious agents are seen.
b The cytological features are nonspecific. However, the location, the cytological features and the age of the animal indicate that aspiration from an occipital haematoma should be the primary consideration.
c Occipital haematomas are not uncommon in young dogs. They are thought to be the result of trauma, but trauma may not be observed in all cases. Benign neglect is the treatment of choice since most of these resolve without intervention.

151 a Two different species of *Demodex* mite are visible.
b The longer mite is the typical follicular mite, *D. canis*. The shorter mite is a *Demodex* species that has recently been found in the stratum corneum (instead of the follicles and sebaceous glands) of the dog. It has been called the 'unnamed short, plump *Demodex* species' by some, although one recent paper described a short mite named *D. cornei*. This mite is similar to *D. gatoi* in the cat in that it inhabits the more superficial skin and may be somewhat contagious, where *D. canis* and *D. cati* are not. Topical treatment with lyme-sulphur has been more effective than daily ivermectin alone. (In the dog a third mite has also been recently described. *D. injai* are longer than *D. canis*, and occupy follicles.)

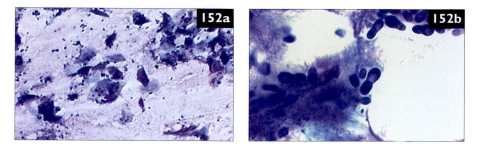

152 You have been treating a five-year-old Newfoundland with otitis externa for several weeks with a topical ear ointment. Because of a poor clinical response you make a few cytological smears from the copious, dark-brown exudate (sweet odour) (152a, b) (Wright–Giemsa, ×10 and ×100 oil, respectively).
a Describe your findings.
b How do you decide whether yeasts are significant or not?
c By what proposed theories does *Malassezia* cause otitis?
d Which special stains can be used to demonstrate *Malassezia*, and what are the staining characteristics with these stains?

153 A six-year-old dog presented with a submandibular swelling. An FNA was collected and a smear prepared.
a What cell types and material are present (153) (Papanicolaou, ×40)?
b What is your diagnosis?

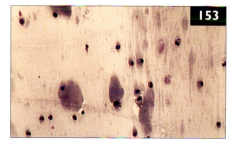

154 Bone marrow aspiration is performed on a dog with pancytopenia with nonregenerative anaemia.
a Describe the cells represented in this photomicrograph (154) (May–Grünwald–Giemsa, ×100).
b What is your diagnosis, and what are the differential diagnoses?

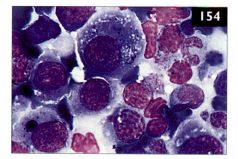

152 a There are large numbers of superficial squamous epithelial cells, squamous debris and very high numbers of broad-based budding structures resembling the sole of a shoe, most compatible with yeast. The most likely differential is *Malassezia pachydermatis* (also known as *Malassezia canis*).
b A diagnosis of mycotic otitis externa is supported by the identification of >10 organisms per ×40 objective, or >4 organisms per oil-immersion field. *Malassezia* is found three times more frequently in otitic ears than in normal ears.
c The inflammation may be due to the by-products of lipid/*Malassezia* interaction (e.g. formation of peroxides) or type I hypersensitivity reaction to *Malassezia* and its by-products.
d Gram's stain: basophilic colour; PAS stain: PAS-positive, bright magenta colour.

153 a Clumps of inspissated purple to pink material consistent with mucus of salivary gland origin. There are a moderate number of nucleated cells that are virtually all foamy, active macrophages.
b The cytological diagnosis is a salivary mucocele. The cytological appearance is characteristic and is the same with Wright–Giemsa or Papanicolaou stains. Mucoid material may vary from moderate to abundant but often occurs in clumps, consistent with some degree of dessication or inspissation. There are usually moderate numbers of foamy, active macrophages. There may be variable numbers of erythrocytes and neutrophils associated with blood contamination, haemorrhage and/or concurrent inflammation. Salivary gland epithelial cells are rarely seen.

154 a The majority of the cells have an obvious histiocytic appearance, but exhibit numerous atypias: coarse chromatin; deeply basophilic cytoplasm in which the clear vacuoles stand out; and high nuclear:cytoplasmic ratio in some cells.
b Diagnosis: malignant histiocytosis (Bernese Mountain Dog). Differential diagnosis: systemic histiocytosis.

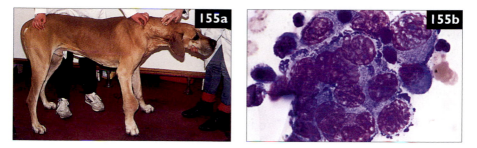

155 A Great Dane (155a) has developed a painful carpal swelling and is lame. An FNA is collected and a smear made (155b) (Wright–Giemsa, ×100 oil).
a What cells are present?
b What is your diagnosis?

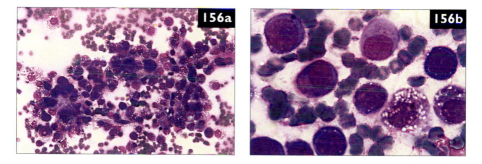

156 An FNA is collected from a canine subcutaneous mass.
a Describe the cells represented in these smears (156a, b) (May–Grünwald–Giemsa, ×25 and ×100 oil, respectively).
b What is your diagnosis, and what are the differential diagnoses?

157 A nine-year-old female Rottweiler is dull and ataxic. A CSF aspirate has an NCC of $0.3 \times 10^9/l$ (normal = $<0.01 \times 10^9/l$) and a TP of 1.7 g/l (normal = <0.6 g/l). A cytospun smear of the fluid is made (157) (Wright–Giemsa, ×100 oil).
a What cells are present?
b What is your diagnosis?

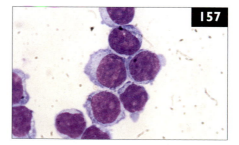

155 a A population of highly pleomorphic cells is seen, with wide variation in nuclear:cytoplasmic ratio. The cytoplasm is deeply basophilic and the nuclei have markedly clumped chromatin. Multinucleated giant cells were seen in other fields.
b In large dogs, tumours at this site are often osteosarcomas. The cytological interpretation is a giant cell tumour of bone.
Note: A giant cell tumour of bone is considered to be a bone tumour that is not a variant of osteosarcoma. Giant cell tumours of bone are uncommon, but have been reported to metastasize. They may appear similar to osteosarcomas in clinical presentation and radiographic appearance.

156 a A highly cellular sample with a haemorrhagic background is shown in **156a**. At high magnification (**156b**) there is a round cell population with a great variation in the nuclear:cytoplasmic ratio: the cells have a round nucleus with a finely stippled chromatin and several poorly visible nucleoli. The cytoplasm varies from grey-blue and vacuolated to deeply basophilic in the less differentiated cell with the highest nuclear:cytoplasmic ratio. However, this population does not demonstrate convincing criteria of malignancy.
b Diagnosis: benign histiocytic granuloma. Differential diagnosis: haematopoietic malignancies (lymphoid or histiocytic).

157 a The cells are an almost homogeneous population of large discrete cells. They have varying amounts of moderately basophilic cytoplasm, sometimes with cytoplasmic projections or pseudopodia. While occasionally irregular, the nuclei are mostly round, with clumped chromatin and one or more prominent nucleoli.
b Lymphosarcoma. This was confirmed on postmortem examination.

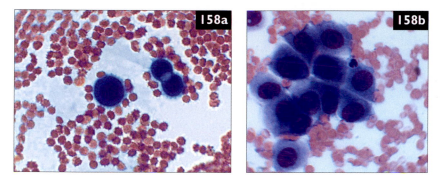

158 A seven-year-old neutered male King Charles Cavalier Spaniel presented with an abdominal effusion.
a Describe the cells you see in these smears (**158a, b**) (Papanicolaou, ×100 oil and Wright–Giemsa, ×100 oil, respectively).
b What is your interpretation of this finding?
c What is the significance of this finding?

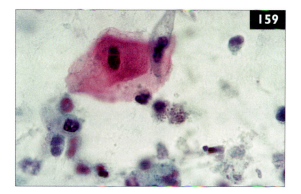

159 A four-year-old Thoroughbred show jumper is referred for evaluation of a chronic cough and possible decreased performance. A tracheal washing is collected by endoscope and submitted for cytological evaluation.
a What cells and structures can you identify in this photomicrograph (**159**) (Papanicolaou, ×100 oil)?
b Other fields in the cytological preparation failed to demonstrate any macrophages or columnar or cuboidal epithelial cells. The features in this photomicrograph are representative of the entire smear. What is your conclusion?

158 a There are a few erythrocytes and single cells and groups of cells with large, oval nuclei and single, distinct nucleoli. The cytoplasm is moderate and faintly granular. The groups of cells are not tightly cohesive. There are 'slits' or 'windows' between the cells. These 'slits' or 'windows' are characteristic of mesothelial cells. A group of epithelial cells would be expected to exhibit tight intercellular junctions without these gaps.

b These cells are consistent with reactive mesothelial cells. In some instances, reactive mesothelial cells may be difficult or impossible to differentiate from malignancy of mesothelial or epithelial origin.

c Because these cells are consistent with a reaction to irritation, they indicate that the effusion has likely been present for at least several days.

159 a There are scattered neutrophils, some of which are outside the plane of focus. There are two large, orange-pink cells with central, small, oval nuclei that are squamous epithelial cells and consistent with oropharyngeal origin. The orange-pink staining of squamous epithelium with the Papanicolaou stain is indicative of the presence of keratohyalin and its precursors. Some small bacterial rods are present in clumps in the centre and upper left.

b In the absence of cells representative of the pulmonary tree (macrophages and columnar or cuboidal epithelial cells), the specimen likely reflects oropharyngeal contamination. The neutrophils may reflect oropharyngeal inflammation. Therefore, the cytological specimen is considered unsatisfactory for evaluation since it lacks cells representative of the lung. Some macrophages and epithelial cells from large (columnar) and/or small airways (cuboidal epithelium and/or macrophages) should be present for tracheal washing to be considered to be satisfactory for evaluation and likely to be representative of the lung.

Oropharyngeal contamination is more likely to occur if the horse is fractious, if the mouth is not washed out prior to collection or if the passage of the endoscope into the trachea is difficult or prolonged. A note to the cytologist indicating whether any of these events has occurred is often helpful in determining if such cells are likely to be due to contamination. If cells representative of the lung are present and oropharyngeal material is also seen, the possibility of oropharyngeal contamination or of abnormal drainage of oropharyngeal material into the trachea in association with a laryngeal or pharyngeal abnormality should be considered. A small amount of oropharyngeal material may be considered to be within expected limits for background contamination. There are skilled collectors who seldom submit endoscopic washings with evidence of oropharyngeal contamination. When oropharyngeal material is present in their specimens, the author always cautions them to consider possible laryngeal or pharyngeal dysfunction in their differential diagnoses. Dynamic evaluation of oropharyngeal and laryngeal function with exercise on the treadmill may be needed in order to diagnosis pharyngeal or laryngeal dysfunction that may contribute to oropharyngeal material draining into the pharynx in some cases.

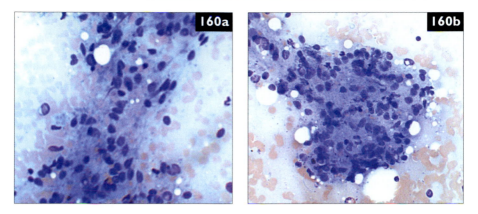

160 Splenomegaly was noted on palpation and ultrasound examination of a 12-year-old neutered female Beagle. A splenic aspirate was collected.
a Describe the features you see in these photomicrographs of the aspirate (**160a, b**) (both Wright–Giemsa, ×50 oil).
b What is your interpretation?
c What is the significance of this finding?

161 An eight-year-old spayed female Akita presented with a chronic cough of four months' duration that had not been responsive to antibiotic therapy. The cough was productive, and the owner reported that the dog frequently coughed up mucus. Radiographs revealed a combined interstitial, alveolar and bronchial pattern. A CBC revealed a moderate eosinophilia (3.4×10^9/l [normal $0.1–1.3 \times 10^9$/l]). A

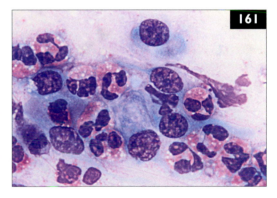

tracheal wash was performed and cytospin preparations made of the material obtained. The microphotograph illustrates a microscopic field representative of the tracheal wash cytology (**161**) (Wright's, ×100).
a What are your differential diagnoses?
b What other diagnostic test(s) do you recommend?

153

160 a There are backgrounds with many erythrocytes, and groups of loosely associated spindle cells with small, uniform oval nuclei containing stippled, evenly distributed chromatin. Nucleoli are small, absent or inconspicuous. The cytoplasm is delicate and wispy and elongated. There are scattered blue-green granules within macrophages that are consistent with haemosiderin.
b A fibrous proliferation with haemosiderin, consistent with splenic hyperplasia.
c This finding may or may not be significant. It likely reflects splenic stimulation but does not reflect an underlying cause.

161 a Allergic and parasitic bronchitis/bronchopneumonitis are the two most likely diagnoses. Fungal elements may also induce an eosinophilic infiltrate.
b Careful examination of multiple slides for parasitic larvae (such as *Oslerus osleri*) is indicated. If none are found, a faecal Baermann's flotation test should be performed as the parasite may be swallowed when the dog coughs up sputum. Bronchoscopic examination may reveal the presence of parasitic nodules at the bifurcation of the trachea with *O. osleri* infection. These may also be observed on radiographs. Allergic bronchitis is diagnosed by exclusion of parasitic infection and a response to corticosteroid therapy, as well as identification of an allergen, if possible, in the animal's environment.
Note: Other less common differential considerations should include the possibility of pulmonary eosinophilic infiltrates, which may be focal. These may be idiopathic or associated with heartworm disease. Some types of tumour (mast cell tumour, T-cell lymphomas or some types of epithelial and mesothelial malignancies) have also been associated with eosinophilic infiltrates, but would be differentiated by localizing clinical signs and histories that vary from that given in this case. It may be very difficult to determine an inciting antigen in cases of allergy to inhaled antigens. In rare cases, food allergy has been implicated as contributing to respiratory clinical signs.

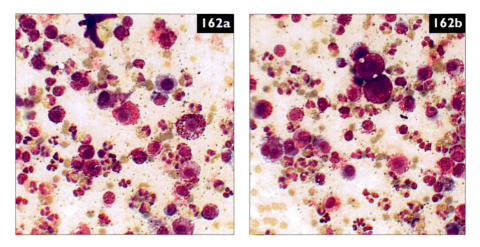

162 A ten-year-old entire male Labrador Retriever presented with multiple skin masses. An aspirate was collected from a mass near the right axilla.
a Describe the features shown in these smears (162a, b) (both Wright–Giemsa, ×50 oil).
b What is your interpretation?
c What are your prognosis and recommendation?

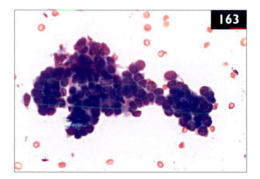

163 An FNA is collected from a mass on the left shoulder of a ten-year-old female neutered DSH cat.
a Describe the cells shown in the smear (163) (Wright–Giemsa ×50 oil).
b What is your interpretation of these findings?
c What prognosis do you expect?

155

162 a There is a moderate number of erythrocytes on a granular background, with a moderate number of eosinophils and a moderate number to many discrete 'round cells' with oval nuclei, some of which can be seen to contain distinct nucleoli. The cytoplasm is oval and varies from faintly or moderately granulated to sparsely or moderately vacuolated. The granules are metachromatic. There are several binucleated cells present, with slight to moderate anisokaryosis amongst the nuclei within a single cell. There is moderate anisocytosis.
b The cytological features are consistent with a poorly differentiated mast cell tumour.
c The prognosis for poorly differentiated mast cell tumours is poor. The presence of multiple masses suggests there may be multiple tumours, which makes the prognosis very poor. Evaluation for possible metastases (usually via regional lymph nodes) is recommended.

163 a There are a few erythrocytes and a lobular group of small cells with relatively uniform, oval nuclei containing finely granular chromatin. Nucleoli are small, absent or inconspicuous. The cytoplasm is scant and homogeneous. Cell boundaries are often indistinct, but nuclei can be seen palisading along the edge (nuclei in a row) of the group in some areas.
b The cytological interpretation is of a basal cell tumour (trichoblastoma). The most common mistake made in the cytological diagnosis of basal cell tumour is that the groups of cells are confused with spindle cells. This is easily done since boundaries are indistinct; sometimes the cytoplasm will appear wispy and the cells are not well-differentiated. Looking for nuclei in a 'row' or palisading along the edge of the groups is a clue to the epithelial origin of these cells.
c With complete removal, the prognosis for a basal cell tumour (trichoblastoma) is usually good. Basal cell tumours in cats may exhibit a range of behaviour from benign to malignant. Usually they are locally invasive but they do not commonly metastasize. There may be some individual tumour cells or small groups of tumour cells at a distance from the macroscopic mass, so generous excision is needed.

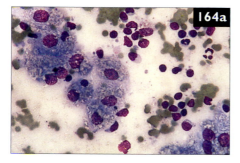

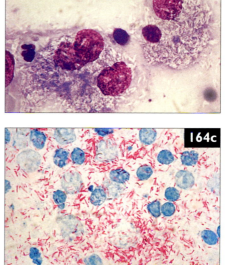

164 An FNA is collected from a feline lymph node.

a Describe the cells represented in these smears (**164a–c**) (May–Grünwald–Giemsa, ×40 and ×100 oil, and Ziehl–Neelsen, ×100 oil, respectively).

b What is your diagnosis and what are the differential diagnoses?

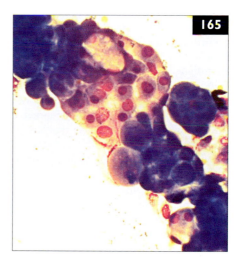

165 A 12-year-old neutered male mixed breed dog presents because of occasional episodes of syncope during exercise. The dog has moderate ascites and chest sounds are masked on auscultation. Radiographs reveal thoracic effusion. Neither chest nor abdominal radiographs show evidence of a mass. Thoracocentesis yields orange-tinged, mildly cloudy fluid (TP = 25 g/l; NCC = 2.7 × 10^9/l). Slides are prepared from material obtained following the cytospin technique.

a What are your differential diagnoses based on the appearance of this smear (**165**) (Wright's, ×100 oil)?

b List any other diagnostic tests you would perform.

157

164 a Clusters of nonphagocytic histiocytes with a foamy cytoplasm among a background of small lymphocytes are seen in **164a**. At high magnification (**164b**) the foamy aspect of the cytoplasm is shown to be due to the presence of numerous clear, slender, elongated intracytoplasmic inclusions. The positive Ziehl–Neelsen-stained smear (**164c**) shows numerous red acid-fast bacilli.
b Diagnosis: mycobacteriosis (*Mycobacterium lepraemurium*). Differential diagnosis: none.

165 a The cells observed are compatible with either malignant glandular epithelial or malignant mesothelial cells. Several nuclear criteria of malignancy are present – anisokaryosis, variable and occasionally high nuclear:cytoplasmic ratio, irregular nuclear shape (nuclear pleomorphism) – as well as nonspecific criteria, including intense cytoplasmic basophilia. On closer examination and in other microscopic fields, additional nuclear criteria of malignancy were observed – nuclear moulding and multiple nucleoli. A mitotic figure is present in the field shown (upper right); this characteristic is not specific for malignancy unless an asymmetric pattern is noted. Although signet ring cells (right and left of centre), cells with a large vacuole that may distend the cell and/or compress the nucleus, suggest glandular epithelial cells, nonmalignant mesothelial cells may demonstrate similar features. Acinar structures, if present (not illustrated), are also suggestive of glandular neoplasia, but this is also a feature that can be observed with mesothelial cells in cytological preparations.
b Additional testing to locate a mass (e.g. ultrasonography) can be done. If imaging results in detection of a mass, ultrasound-guided aspiration can be attempted. Exploratory laparotomy and biopsy would enable histological examination. In some cases, further testing such as immunocytochemistry or electron microscopy is required to distinguish definitively between a poorly differentiated carcinoma and mesothelioma.
Note: The differentiation of malignant from reactive mesothelial cells and of mesothelial malignancy from adenocarcinoma are classic dilemmas in cytology.

Mesothelial cells are characterized ultrastructurally by the presence of numerous microvilli, which are not seen in cells of adenocarcinoma. The microvillous surface is often reflected in Papanicolaou-stained smears as a peripheral that stains less densely and has a ruffled appearance; this has been compared to a 'petticoat' but may not be apparent in malignant mesothelial cells. In Romanowsky-stained smears this 'petticoat' may appear as a 'hairy' or 'sunburst' border. Vacuolation in mesothelial cells may mimic secretory vacuoles of adenocarcinoma. Staining with Mucicarmine or Alcian Blue-PAS may be helpful, since secretion will stain red to pink, respectively. Secretion is not present in mesothelial cells and vacuolation may represent a degenerative or reactive change.

Sometimes patterns of articulation of cells will be helpful in differentiating mesothelial cells from those of epithelial origin. In groups of mesothelial cells there may be spaces between adjacent cells, referred to as 'clefts', 'windows' or 'slits' by various authors, that are not typically seen at junctions between epithelial cells. Tissue fragments of mesothelial cells may have a central core of collagen that is not usually present with epithelial configurations unless large papillary extensions break off into the fluid of a body cavity. Tissue fragments of mesothelial cells also may have a knobbly appearance with individual cells protruding from the periphery of groups; this appearance is not commonly seen in groups of epithelial origin. Multinucleation and mitotic figures may occur in either proliferative, nontumerous mesothelial cells, malignant mesothelial cells or epithelial cells, so they are not useful in differentiating these cell types or processes.

Finally, mesothelial cells in washings of body cavities, or cells that have been collected in large animals (cows, horses) using a large bore needle or teat cannula, may exfoliate as medium to large, flat groups of cells with a mosaic appearance. This appearance is usually attributed to mechanical exfoliation without the natural exfoliation into fluid that results in 'rounding up' of the cells. Such groups have occasionally been seen exfoliated in horses with abdominal thromboembolism associated with colic (presumably resulting in hypoxic exfoliation), but without apparent traumatic exfoliation.

Frequently asked questions

FAQ1   How can cytology be of value to me in practice?

Cytology can be of value in determining a diagnosis, a type of process and/or possible differential diagnoses. It may be of benefit for prognosis, treatment planning (including surgical or medical approach) and client education. It may also be of benefit for monitoring the progression of conditions or determining response to treatment.

When the use of cytology is being contemplated, the following should be considered:

- The value of cytology lies in its ability to affect the progress or handling of a case in a manner that would not have been possible had cytology not been done.
- If the use of cytology does not have the potential to affect your approach or handling of a case, its use is questionable.
- If cytology does not consistently provide a high degree of useful, accurate information, it is of questionable value.

FAQ2   When should I use cytology in practice, and when should I submit specimens to a specialist cytology service?

The following points should be considered:

- Is my time best used for this purpose (cytological evaluation) or for other techniques? Need to consider economics, customer service and existing needs within your practice.
- Do I have sufficient training, practice and interest consistently to obtain specimens of diagnostic quality?
- Do I have sufficient interest and training, or time, to devote to training, in order to prepare and stain specimens of diagnostic quality and to have reasonable confidence in my interpretations?
- Do I have a good quality microscope to use? (See also **FAQ14**)
- What is the availability of a cytologist/cytopathologist? Do I have a good relationship with a cytologist/cytopathologist whom I trust and like?

Reasons to have cytology preparations and stains available, whether or not you use a cytologist/cytopathologist's services include:

- Confirmation of cellularity of the specimen and likely adequacy of collection, enabling repeated sampling if few or no cells are identified.
- Ability to report preliminary results to owner if immediately prepared.
- Enhance learning of cytological interpretation by comparison with cytologist/cytopathologist's results.
- Enhance clinical investigative abilities and differential diagnoses by comparison of clinical considerations and cytological results.

Good reasons for using a cytologist/cytopathologist's services include:

- External confirmation of clinical suspicions and concerns.
- Utilization of expertise and training of a specialist in cytological evaluation.
- Provision of 'added value' to client service (i.e. consultation with a specialist).
- Possible availability of special stains, concentrating techniques, immunological staining, etc. that may aid in diagnosis and/or prognosis.

FAQ3   What is considered essential for a good cytology preparation?

Essentials for good cytology preparations include:

Appropriate collection materials and/or devices:

- Usually a 21–25 gauge needle and 5–10 ml syringe are appropriate for fine needle aspiration of cutaneous masses or lesions or body fluids.
- A tuberculin or 25 gauge needle without a syringe is suitable for needle sampling without aspiration. Particularly beneficial for superficial lesions or samples that may exhibit increased cellular fragility, such as enlarged lymph nodes.
- Special holders or devices may be of benefit in improving dexterity and cellularity of specimens.
- Scalpel blades of varying sizes and types may be needed for scrapings.
- Swabs should be dampened with saline or transport medium prior to cell collection in order to prevent dehydration and distortion of cells.
- Some specimens (e.g. bone marrow and CSF) require special needles with a stylet.

(Continued overleaf)

(FAQ3 continued)

Clean, high quality slides:

- Oil residue can be removed by immersion in alcohol and wiping with lint-free tissue.
- Frosted end slides preferred for ease of labelling and identification.
- If volume permits, multiple slides are preferred in order to increase probability of representative specimen.
- Keep slides covered to prevent accumulation of dust and other air-borne material.

Rapid air drying (hair dryer is useful):

- Prevents 'balling up' of cells that hinders identification and evaluation of nuclear and cytoplasmic features.
- Rapid air drying promotes optimal cell spreading, prevention of artefacts and adherence to the slide.

Problem-solving techniques:

- If the specimen is highly viscous and difficult to spread, consider expulsion of material into a small drop of serum prior to smearing.
- Anticoagulant (usually EDTA or sodium citrate) should be available in case bloody specimens or specimens that clot are obtained on initial attempt.

Suitable tubes or holders for transport and submission of specimens:

- Fixative (40% ethanol or 10% buffered formalin) may be suitable for some types of specimens and if appropriate staining techniques (e.g. Papanicolaou, H & E, New Methylene Blue) are used.
- Slide holders should be used to protect smears from dust and dirt and to prevent breakage.
- Protect air-dried smears from formalin fumes that may interfere with staining by Romanowsky methods.

FAQ4   How should I collect cytology specimens?

Fine needle aspirate
Advantages:
- Suitable for sampling many types of cutaneous masses or lesions.
- Usually does not require sedation or anaesthesia. Minimal sedation or anaesthesia may be required in special cases.

Disadvantages:
- Certain types of lesions may exfoliate poorly on aspiration, especially fibrotic lesions or some tumours of mesenchymal origin.
- Overenthusiastic aspiration may result in blood contamination or haemodilution.

Technique:
- 21–25 gauge needle and 5–10 ml syringe usually adequate.
- Redirect multiple times within the mass in order to increase probability of representative specimen.
- Discontinue suction prior to withdrawal.
- Detach syringe and draw in several millilitres of air.
- Reattach syringe to needle and gently expel material onto labelled glass slides.
- Smear and air dry rapidly (hair dryer).

Ultra-fine needle sampling without aspiration
Advantages:
- Preserves morphology of fragile cells.
- Minimizes or eliminates blood contamination and haemodilution.
- Particularly good for superficial masses and those that may contain fragile cells such as lymph nodes.

Disadvantages:
- Not suitable for deep lesions.
- Not suitable for lesions that exfoliate poorly without aspiration.

Technique:
- Tuberculin or 25 gauge needle usually used.
- 'Stick' mass several times and in multiple areas to obtain a 'core' of representative cells within the needle.
- May see material within hub of needle.
- Withdraw needle.
- Attach syringe containing several millilitres of air.
- Gently expel material onto labelled glass slides.
- Smear and air dry rapidly (hair dryer).

(Continued overleaf)

(FAQ4 continued)

Scraping
Advantages:
- Appropriate for identification of mites and ringworm.
- Some types of lesions that may exfoliate poorly may be adequately sampled by scraping.
- Suitable for ulcerated lesions.

Disadvantages:
- Requires relatively 'deep' scraping to increase probability of representative cells and not just exudate associated with an ulcer.
- May be prone to 'thick' areas containing poorly separated cells that are difficult to interpret.

Technique:
- Use sterile scalpel blade.
- Smear material on labelled glass slide(s).
- Can make 'squash' preparation to facilitate separation of cells.
- Thin spreads may be facilitated by addition of small amount of serum.
- Air dry rapidly (hair dryer).

Imprints
Advantages:
- Usually low probability of information unless done from cut surface of a biopsy.
- Tend to represent surface inflammation, haemorrhage and/or contamination without inclusion of material representative of deeper cells and processes.
- May be useful for demonstration of superficial yeast (*Malassezia*) or organisms (usually bacteria).

Disadvantage:
- Not appropriate for most ulcerated or nonulcerated masses.

Technique:
- Gentle wiping with gauze may be of benefit in removing superficial crust or debris that would prevent exfoliation of underlying cells.
- Gently touch surface of labelled slide to area of interest.
- If abundant material is obtained, a 'squash' preparation is suitable. If only a small amount of material, no additional smearing is needed.
- Air dry rapidly (hair dryer).
- Examination of crusts and superficial material may be of benefit in identifying some types of processes.

Swab

Advantages:
- Appropriate for evaluation of exudates or exploration of sinus tracts or draining lesions.
- May be helpful in obtaining material from vesicles or pustules.

Disadvantage:
- Not appropriate for most ulcerated or nonulcerated masses.

Technique:
- Dampen swab with sterile saline or transport medium prior to collection in order to prevent cell dehydration, lysis and distortion.
- Gently roll swab along slide to dislodge cells.
- Air dry rapidly (hair dryer).

'Scratch and sniff' preparations from biopsies

Advantages:
- May provide more representative material than imprints.
- Useful for rapid evaluation and for 'learning' cytology from corresponding histological description and diagnosis.

Disadvantages:
- Best preparations obtained from unfixed tissue (suitable for Romanowsky stains) or tissue that has not been in formalin >12 hours (suitable for Papanicolaou, Trichrome and H&E stains or wet mounts).
- Cells obtained from tissue in fixative for longer periods of time may not adhere to glass slide, may 'ball up' or may not stain optimally, depending on stain type used.

Technique:
- Identify likely representative area of biopsy.
- Sample from several areas to increase probability of representative cells.
- Use one corner of a clean slide to gently 'scratch' the surface of the biopsy.
- Transfer material from corner of the slide to another slide surface.
- 'Squash' preparations are usually best.
- If rubbery consistency or poor spreading, addition of a small amount of serum may facilitate making thin spreads.
- Air dry rapidly (hair dryer) if Romanowsky stains to be used.
- Treat appropriately if other stains are to be used.

(Continued overleaf)

(FAQ4 continued)

Washing or lavage
Advantages:
- May provide collection from a wide area or from tubular organs such as lung or reproductive tract.
- May be more sensitive than swab or focal collections.

Disadvantage:
- Requires careful definition of 'adequacy' or 'representativeness' of specimens.

Technique:
- Varies with site and/or species.
- See literature and textbooks for descriptions of washing and lavage collection.

Aspiration of body fluids
Advantages:
- Suitable for abdominal fluid, pleural fluid, pericardial fluid, synovial fluid and CSF.
- May provide therapeutic advantage by removal of excess fluid.
- May provide information about processes shedding diagnostic cells or elements into body fluids.

Disadvantage:
- May not reflect pathological processes, resulting in excess fluid accumulation.

Technique:
- Varies with site and/or species.
- See literature and textbooks for descriptions of collection technique.

FAQ5   How should I prepare my cytology specimens?

A variety of methods can be used depending on the type of specimen and the cellularity. A summary of the type of presentation, techniques and comments regarding the presentations is shown below.

Direct smears. Suitable for most aspirates of cutaneous masses. Concentration of cells may be needed for specimens of low cellularity.

Blood smear technique
Technique:
- Same as that used for blood smear preparation.
- Drop of specimen is placed at one end of slide.
- Pull end of second slide into the drop at an approximately 45° angle.
- Push portion of drop toward the end of the slide to create a smear that extends approximately three-quarters of the length of slide and which has a feather edge.

Comments:
- Blood smear technique is appropriate for bloody specimens, specimens that are predominantly 'liquid' or specimens that can be expelled into a small drop of serum.
- Larger cells or cell clumps are likely to be concentrated at edges of smear and along feather edge.
- Use of a 'spreader slide' with rounded or angled corners is helpful in producing a smear that is slightly narrower than the width of the slide.
- Spreader slide should be cleaned carefully after use to remove any residual cells and prevent accumulation of dried material that may cause uneven spreading of cell film.

'Pull apart' smears or 'squash' preparations
Technique:
- This technique is the one preferred by the author for most direct smears.
- Material is gently expelled onto a slide.
- A second slide is placed on top of the first slide and its weight is allowed to spread or 'squash' the material.
- The slides are slid apart or 'pulled apart', resulting in cells smeared on both slides.
- Smears should not travel over the edge of the slide and should not be too close to the edge of the slide.

Comments:
- Care should be taken to prevent excessive pressure on the top slide; this may result in rupture or smudging of cells.
- Some types of rubbery specimens or specimens that are of thick consistency may benefit from expulsion into a small drop of serum to aid the spreading.
- Gentle circular motions of the top slide may help 'break up' or spread thick accumulations of material or cells.
- Excessive dilution by serum, fluid or blood may result in migration of cells to the edges of the slide. Carefully observe spreading of droplet to prevent loss of cells.

(Continued overleaf)

(FAQ5 continued)

'Line' smears
Technique:
- These smears are made in the same way as the blood smear technique, but instead of completing the smear to form a feather edge, the spreader slide is lifted vertically prior to formation of a feather edge. This results in concentration of cells along a 'line' where the smear is interrupted.

Comment:
- Suitable for the same types of specimens as for blood smear technique.

'Star' spreads
Technique:
- This is the author's 'least favourite' method of presentation but it can produce nice presentations when done expertly.
- Material is expelled onto a slide as a droplet.
- A needle or syringe cap is drawn through the droplet in a configuration like that of drawing a five- or six-pointed star.
- This produces a central thick area with thinner 'arms' of the star radiating from it.

Comments:
- Suitable for fluid specimens or for specimens for which the blood smear technique can be used.
- Often results in the majority of cells remaining in the central 'thick' area; may be impossible or difficult to evaluate.
- Rapid air drying is more difficult to achieve due to the uneven thickness of the preparation.

Indirect smears. These types of preparations require concentration of cells. Suitable for specimens of low cellularity, specimens in which there is blood or other fluid components or specimens that are added to a small volume of sterile bacterial transport medium or saline containing 10% serum.

Centrifugation
Technique:
- Gentle centrifugation of specimens that are fluid, contain blood or have been added to a small quantity of sterile bacterial transport medium or saline containing 10% serum is used to concentrate cells in a pellet at the bottom of the tube.
- Centrifugation equipment and speeds as used for urinalysis and/or separation of serum are appropriate for cell concentration.
- Supernatant is decanted or aspirated.
- Cells are resuspended in a small amount of the fluid remaining in the tube or are aspirated directly from the pellet using a small, disposable pipette.
- The cell suspension droplet is transferred to a slide.
- A smear is made by spreading the material with the pipette or by a 'pull apart' or 'squash' technique, depending on the amount of material that is present.

Comments:
- Use of conical tubes facilitates pelleting of sample and easy retention of cells following supernatant decanting. Cells can be resuspended in the small amount of fluid remaining after decanting.
- Concentration by centrifugation is helpful for specimens of low cellularity that may not be easily evaluated in a direct smear preparation.
- If no 'pellet' of cells is visible following centrifugation, special concentration techniques should be considered.

Special concentration techniques
- Special concentration techniques are not likely to be available in most practices. They are more commonly available in large referral practices or in laboratories that specialize in cytological preparations.
- Special concentration techniques that may be encountered include cytocentrifugation, membrane filtration techniques, thin-prep techniques and/or sedimentation chambers.

FAQ6   What stains should I use for cytology specimens?

The stains commonly used for cytology specimens are:

> **Romanowsky stains:**
> - Diff-Quik. NB: Stains some mast cell granules in mast cell tumours very poorly.
> - Wright-Giemsa.
> - Other Quik stains.
>
> **Wet mounts:**
> - New Methylene Blue
>
> **Stains requiring wet-fixation:**
> - Papanicolaou or Trichrome (some rehydration protocols described for use with air-dried smears).
> - Haematoxylin and Eosin (H&E).
>
> **Commonly used 'special stains':**
> - Gram's stain for gram-negative and gram-positive bacteria.
> - Ziehl-Neelsen (acid-fast) stain for acid-fast bacteria.
> - Prussian Blue stain for iron.

Romanowsky stains are those most commonly used in practice. There are a number of rapid stains, of which Diff-Quik is the most well known. Consistency in application and standardization of staining times are important for achieving good quality, consistent results. Take the time to try several different timings in order to pick the one with the best nuclear and cytoplasmic contrast. Be prepared to stain lymph node aspirates and bone marrow aspirates for approximately twice the time used for fluids or routine aspirates. Try the routine timing and see if the stain is adequate. If not, the smears can be run through the stain again in an attempt to achieve better staining.

Stain maintenance is an important part of quality control and ensuring that consistent results are obtained.

Stain maintenance and quality control:
- Protect from sunlight.
- Keep covered when not in use.
- Filter periodically (coffee filters are an inexpensive source and acceptable for most stains).
- Clean jars frequently to prevent accumulation of precipitate, growth of organisms and 'floaters' (cells or organisms that may be within stain and 'float' onto and adhere to a smear; not a true reflection of the lesion, but may contribute to misdiagnosis).
- Replace stains as indicated by storage, volume of smears and other conditions.
- Know the stain and its capabilities with regard to colours, transparency and differentiation.
- Standardize staining times and procedures.
- Know possible artefacts produced by ageing of the stain.
- Know possible artefacts produced by nonadherence to standard operating procedures.
- Can use buccal smears (cells scraped from the inside of your cheek) as control smears periodically to evaluate staining adequacy, quality and technique.
- Know the 'contaminants' associated with your practice: leave slide on bench top during the day and/or overnight in order to accumulate air-borne contaminants.

FAQ7 **What are the advantages and disadvantages of using a stain for fixed specimens (e.g. Papanicolaou, Sano's modification of Pollack's Trichrome or Haematoxylin and Eosin)?**

These stains are traditionally used on fixed specimens. Fixation is helpful in preventing cellular degeneration, metabolism and maturation and in preventing bacterial overgrowth *in vitro*. The nuclear detail provided by these stains is superior because it uses haematoxylin (the same stain as used on tissue sections). The staining characteristics and hues differ from traditional Romanowsky stains and may require experience to identify subtle changes. Bacteria may be more difficult to identify than in Romanowsky-stained smears, particularly when present in small numbers. There are some rapid versions of these stains available, but Romanowsky stains are more commonly used in private practice. These stains may be available in some commercial laboratories. Check with your preferred reference laboratory for the possible availability of these stains and techniques.

FAQ8   What should I expect or include in a cytology report?

The format for a cytology report can vary between laboratories and according to individuals' preferences. The commonly encountered sections of a cytology report are listed below:

Summary of clinical information:
- May or may not be included.
- In the author's opinion it is useful to summarize pertinent clinical information about the case.

Description:
- May or may not include macroscopic features (colour, transparency, character and macroscopic content).
- Should include microscopic features.
- Even if pathologists disagree in the interpretation of findings, the description should be similar!

Interpretation:
- Diagnosis or differential diagnoses.
- Degree of confidence in interpretation.

Comments:
- Aetiology (if identifiable).
- Prognosis.
- Client education (e.g. expected biological behaviour).
- Address questions or aspects of clinical significance.
- Include other tests or procedures that may be helpful in obtaining a more definitive diagnosis, further definition of the condition and/or planning for treatment (e.g. T and B cell immunophenotyping, serology, bone marrow aspiration, clinical chemistry, etc).
- Monitoring that may be appropriate (e.g. regional lymph nodes, local recurrence, multiple tumours).
- Other recommendations (treatment considerations [if knowledgeable], etc).

FAQ9   What types of cytology specimens should be referred to an experienced cytologist?

The following should be considered for referral to an experienced cytologist:
- All specimens (?).
- Specimens about which you have a question.
- Inflammatory lesions that have not responded to treatment.
- For a second opinion in cases that have a poor prognosis or unusual or unexpected findings.

FAQ10 If a cytology specimen does not provide good information or is not representative, is it worth repeating?

In many instances an initial unsatisfactory specimen or nonspecific findings may be due to the nature of the lesion. Some types of lesion exfoliate poorly on aspiration or may result in nonspecific features. However, in general, evaluation of additional collections may be helpful in:

- Increasing the probability of detection and/or diagnosis of abnormality.
- Increasing the confidence in interpretation if persistent and/or progressive features are identified.
- Increasing the confidence in negative findings, if repeatable.

FAQ11 How do I know if I have a suitable or satisfactory specimen for interpretation, and that it is representative of the lesion?

This is a question that plagues all cytologists. The suitability of a specimen for interpretation will depend on the type of lesion aspirated. General guidelines for various types of cytological specimen are shown below:

Fine needle aspirates of skin masses or internal masses:
- Usually considered satisfactory/suitable for interpretation if nucleated cells are present. A specimen that does not contain nucleated cells is unsatisfactory or inconclusive.
- Some types of lesion are characterized by low cellularity (e.g. lipomas); other types of lesion (often of mesenchymal origin) may exfoliate poorly on aspiration.

Lymph node aspirate:
- Should contain cells of lymphoid origin.
- Sometimes, a lymph node will be totally effaced by inflammation or malignancy. In cases in which lymphoid cells are not present, lymph node involvement cannot be confirmed or ruled out.

(Continued overleaf)

(FAQ11 continued)

Tracheal or bronchial washing
- Must have cells from several levels of the respiratory tract (columnar and/or cuboidal epithelial cells; macrophages) to have confidence in representation of all levels of the lung.
- Sometimes a limited interpretation is possible if an abnormality is recognized despite the absence of cells from several levels of the lung.

Bronchoalveolar lavage
- Macrophages need to be present in order to be considered representative of small airways and alveoli.
- Other cell types may be present.

Urine
- The absence of cells may be within normal limits.
- 'No abnormality detected' is the most common interpretation when no cells or infectious agents are present.

Cerebrospinal fluid
- The absence of cells may be within normal limits.
- 'No abnormality detected' is the most common interpretation when no cells or infectious agents are present.

Synovial fluid
- Some cells are expected. Normally expect a few small lymphocytes, macrophages and synoviocytes.
- Sometimes other cell types may predominate, depending on the condition that is present.

Pleural and abdominal fluid
- Some cells expected. Normally expect a mixture of neutrophils, macrophages and lymphocytes.
- Sometimes other cell types may predominate, depending on the condition that is present.

Bone marrow aspirate
- Marrow particles and haematopoietic precursors are needed for optimal interpretation.
- Limited interpretation may be possible if some haematopoietic cells are present, even without marrow particles.

Uterine washing
- Normally expect epithelial cells. Rare neutrophils and macrophages may be within normal limits. Epithelial morphology differs, depending on the stage of reproductive activity.
- Sometimes other cell types are present, depending on the condition that is present.

Vaginal smears
- Epithelial cells expected. Bacteria (normal flora) may or may not be present.
- Sometimes other cell types are present, depending on the condition that is present.

Representativeness of a specimen may be difficult to determine. If expected cell types are present in various types of specimen (see above), then there is a high probability that the specimen is representative of the organ or system from which it was obtained. Other factors that need to be taken into account in evaluating whether or not a specimen is likely to be representative of the site of collection include:

- Degree of cellularity.
- Numbers, types and proportions of cells.
- A bloody specimen may complicate the interpretation of many types of specimen.
- Correlation with the clinical appearance and clinical suspicions about the type of lesion.
- Correlation with the location of the lesion and its suspected significance (e.g. tumour metastatic to lymph node).
- Quality of the specimen (cell preservation and staining).

FAQ12 What if the cytological evaluation does not fit with the clinical findings or histological interpretation?

In most cases the cytological findings will correlate well with the clinical findings and histological evaluation. It is imperative that the cytological appearance must be correlated with the clinical picture. If it does NOT fit:

- Use good judgement.
- Contact the cytologist for review or send the specimen to an experienced cytologist for a second opinion.
- Consider additional specimens.

Remember, cytological/histological correlation is expected with cancer. The degree of correlation may vary with noncancerous conditions. Cytology may vary from histology in representation of cell types and degree of abnormality. The sensitivity, specificity, predictive value of cytology and histology may vary with site, type of collection and type of process.

FAQ13 How should I go about evaluating a cytology smear?

The cytological evaluation should be done in a systematic manner, conducted in the same way each time a slide or set of slides is examined. Initially, the smear should be examined at a low magnification, with special attention at the feather edge (if present), along the edges of the smear and within the smear to detect unusual features, cells or groups of cells that may need subsequent examination at a higher magnification.

The low magnification examination will provide information about the overall cellularity and content of the smear and may be helpful in assessing adequacy and representativeness of the specimen, the presentation and staining. Intermediate magnification is used for the major part of the evaluation to help identify various cell types, their proportions and their features. High magnification is used to determine fine detail. Additional screening of the smear at low or intermediate magnification, using overlapping fields to cover the entire slide rapidly, may be needed in some cases.

When a cytological specimen is evaluated, the thought processes of expert evaluators may evolve along different lines, depending on their experience, their training and their mental organization. However, the following thought processes are identified by most expert evaluators:

- Is the specimen adequate for evaluation? Are the presentation and staining quality adequate?
- Is the specimen likely to be representative of the process or condition in question based on the information about lesion appearance, lesion location, method of collection and any problems described with that collection (i.e. likely blood contamination)?
- Is the cellularity sufficient for this type of specimen and method of collection?
- Is there any noncellular or background material that may be of significance (i.e. matrix material produced by some mesenchymal tumours, secretory material, necrotic debris that may indicate 'tumour diathesis', lymphoglandular bodies supporting lymphoid tissue origin, cytoplasmic material that may be secretion or phagocytosed material, etc)?
- What numbers, types and proportions of cells are present?
- Is there a special population of cells that differs from that expected or which should not be present?
- What type of process does this likely represent (i.e. inflammatory, noninflammatory, proliferative, non-neoplastic, neoplastic, benign or malignant)?
- Can the process be further characterized or subcategorized in a way that will provide useful information (i.e. what type of inflammation; if neoplastic, with what type of tumour or group of tumours is this compatible)?
- Is an aetiology apparent (infectious agent, foreign material)?
- If neoplastic, do the cells have features of being benign or malignant?
- If neoplastic, can the cell type of origin be identified specifically or to a particular group or category?
- What degree of confidence is there in the cytological interpretation of the specimen?
- What is the expected biological behaviour based on these findings?
- Are there additional tests that may be of benefit for confirmation, prognosis, staging or evaluation of the extent of the disease?
- Are there treatments or other recommendations that the cytologist is knowledgeable enough to make about this condition?
- Is there a need for a second opinion or additional research into this case (comparison with cases of known diagnoses, literature search, reference text, etc)?

FAQ14 What kind of microscope is the best to use for cytology evaluations?

In general, a binocular microscope is best. The lenses should include low, medium and high magnifications, usually 4, ×10, ×20 and ×40, or ×50 oil and ×100 oil. An adjustable light source and condenser should be present in order to provide the appropriate lighting and contrast that are needed at various magnifications and for a variety of specimens.

FAQ15 What is the best way of preserving slides for an archive?

Slides should be stored in a clean, dry environment and protected from light. In order to prevent damage to the surface of the smear, it should be mounted with a coverslip using a mounting medium such as Permount or Eukitt. These are usually xylene-soluble, and xylene can be used to clean oil from the surface of the smear if it has been examined prior to coverslipping. The coverslip should be mounted without air bubbles and allowed to dry flat before storing. The stored slides should be labelled with indelible marker so that they can be identified for future reference. Slides with a frosted end are particularly useful, since they can be written on in pencil and the pencil will not rub off with storage. A file containing reports or other information corresponding to the smears is useful. Any follow-up information (clinical or histological) can be included in this file.

FAQ16 How often are infectious agents seen in cytological specimens?

The frequency with which infectious agents are seen in cytological specimens will depend on the types of specimens obtained and the conditions most frequently seen in the practice. The absence of infectious agents cytologically does not rule out the possibility of infection. A common cytology teaching adage is: 'the absence of evidence is not evidence of absence'. However, when infections are present, the likelihood of detecting infectious agents is increased when:

- A representative specimen is obtained.
- The specimen is well stained.
- The specimen is examined by a person experienced in the recognition of a variety of infectious agents.

The possibility of false-positive identification of infectious agents also exists. Sometimes, granular precipitate or debris resembles bacteria. If an unfixed specimen is received by post, there may be overgrowth of bacteria from contamination or overgrowth of a pathogen. If fluid specimens are obtained, making a cytological preparation from the freshly collected specimen with minimal or no delay prior to processing is likely to provide the best sample. If referral laboratories offer special stains for fixed specimens (e.g. Papanicolaou, Sano's modification of Pollack's Trichrome stain, H&E or a wet mount preparation using New Methylene Blue), then addition of fixative may help prevent or limit bacterial overgrowth during transport to the laboratory. This is particularly important for specimens that may require overnight transport by post or courier. The availability of such stains for fixed specimens will vary with the laboratory. Fixation will also help preserve cellular morphology and prevent the ongoing degeneration, metabolism or maturation that may occur in unfixed specimens during transport to the laboratory. Check with your referral laboratory for their preferred methods.

The other measures that may be helpful in preventing contamination with infectious agents that would result in false-positive results are:

- Handle specimens only in a clean environment.
- Wash all glassware, pipettes and other instruments frequently. Disposable plastic pipettes are most often used to prevent contamination that may occur when pipettes are reused.
- Place fluid specimens only in clean tubes.
- Do not leave slides in an unprotected environment that may result in environmental contamination of the slide surface.
- Filter stains frequently and make sure that glassware containing stains is clean and free from precipitate and 'floating material'.
- If it known that a specimen probably contains infectious agents or numerous bacteria or yeast, or if other infectious agents are observed on microscopic examination, filter the stains prior to running other slides through the stain.

A standard coffee filter can be used to filter most cytological stains. These filters can be reused until such time as they accumulate sufficient material to block the pores and prevent the liquid from coming through the filter. Remember to filter stain only into a clean, dry jar.

If infectious agents are suspected in some types of preparations (e.g. wet-mounts or unstained urine sediment), then evaluation of a stained sediment smear may be helpful to confirm this suspicion. The presence of intracellular bacteria provides good support for the presence of sepsis. Extracellular bacteria may also indicate infection, but contaminants or overgrowth should also be considered when extracellular organisms are present.

FAQ17 What if my smears stain too darkly (so darkly that I can't identify the cells)?

Smears stained too darkly may be due to:
- Excessively thick smears that are not rapidly air-dried. This may cause cells to round up (not spread out well) and stain very darkly. Hint: a hand-held hair drier or warming plate may be used on a low setting to help dry smears rapidly.
- Excessive staining times in one or more of the solutions with manual staining.
- Presence of excessive mucus or other secretion that may obscure cells and/or contribute to slow air drying.

FAQ18 What do I do if my smears stain very blue, without much contrast between nucleus and cytoplasm?

> **Excessive blue staining may be due to:**
> - Excessive time in the blue stain or too little time in the red/orange stain if using a manual stain. Check that the red/orange stain has not been exhausted when it appears that the staining time is within the expected limits.
> - Exposure to formalin fumes.
> - Incorrect pH of the stains or water.

FAQ19 What should I do if the smear is obscured by clumps of stain precipitate?

> - Filter the stains. Be sure to filter into a clean jar.
> - Clean out the staining jars (use 3% bleach solution to remove any stubborn precipitate staining).
> - Make sure that smears are being rinsed properly. If tap water is used, make sure it is not excessively hard water (may need to use distilled water or a water softener on the water supply).

FAQ20 What should I do if my lymph node and bone marrow aspirates, in particular, stain very pale?

These types of preparation may need adjustments to the staining times. If doing manual staining, you may need to lengthen the staining times (double or triple). If using an automatic stainer, you may want to run the slides through the stainer twice. This may help improve the quality of the staining, but will not be effective for all slides. Sometimes, a wet preparation (can be done on top of the poorly stained smear) with a drop of New Methylene Blue under a coverslip will be helpful. However, sometimes you just have to do the best you can with the pale staining!

FAQ21 What classification should be used for pleural and abdominal fluid specimens, and how is it helpful?

The classical approach to classification of pleural and abdominal fluid specimens is to use nucleated cell count (NCC) and total protein (TP) to determine if the fluid is likely to be a transudate, a modified transudate or an exudate. Other classifications may be based on the cytological findings, including haemorrhagic effusions, neoplastic effusions, nonspecific effusions, pyothorax, pyoabdomen or septic effusions. All classification schemes have drawbacks, since there are some specimens that do not fit nicely into the various classifications provided. The traditional classification system based on NCCs and TP may provide a good starting point for consideration of those conditions that commonly cause these findings. The cytological appearance may or may not provide a likely cause, but it can help determine the best approach for continued investigation or treatment of the condition.

Transudates are classically associated with hypoproteinaemia/hypoalbuminaemia. Usually, albumin is <15–18 g/l before effusion will form due to decreased osmotic colloidal pressure alone. Transudates may also be seen with early cardiac insufficiency or other noninflammatory causes of effusions.

Exudates are most often seen with inflammatory or infectious conditions, but may also occur with neoplastic or lymphocytic effusions that are the result of lymph stasis. Lymph stasis may be associated with cardiac insufficiency or the presence of an internal mass or chylous effusion that is interfering with venous/lymphatic return.

Modified transudates are effusions with intermediate characteristics that may include a variety of underlying causes. The prognosis for these conditions is often poor, since modified transudates are often associated with malignancy or conditions involving organs or systems that are not easily resolved.

FAQ22 What should I do if all I get is a very bloody specimen (effusion or aspirate)?

- Make a buffy coat smear to try to concentrate the nucleated cells. The procedure for making a buffy coat smear is as follows:
- Fill several microhaematocrit tubes with a well-mixed specimen and spin as you would to obtain a PCV.
- With a file, score just BELOW the buffy coat (whitish layer on top of the RBC column).
- Carefully break the tube and gently tap to expel the buffy coat onto a slide. If the material does not come out of the tube with gentle tapping, an unbent paper clip can be inserted into the tube to push the material out gently and onto a slide.
- Make a 'squash preparation' or blood smear type preparation.
- Rapidly air dry.
- Stain with a Romanowsky stain.

Remember that the leukocytes will be numerous in this type of preparation. Platelets (if present) will also be concentrated. Examine carefully for haemic and nonhaemic cell types.

FAQ23 What are the cytological criteria for malignancy?

The following criteria are commonly associated with malignancy. Each by itself, or in some combination, may occur with stimulation of cells associated with hyperplasia or dysplasia or in some cases with inflammation. If the criteria are consistently present and multiple criteria are present, then malignancy is more likely. The criteria include:

- Uneven chromatin distribution.
- Increased chromatin clumping or prominence.
- Nucleoli or macronucleoli (volume of the nucleolus is more than or equal to 50% of the volume of the nucleus) – may be single or multiple.
- Irregularly shaped (not round) nucleoli.
- Increased nuclear:cytoplasmic ratio.
- Mitotic figures, especially if asymmetrical.
- Multinucleation.
- Abnormal variation in cellular size (anisocytosis).
- Abnormal variation in nuclear size (anisokaryosis).
- Inappropriate cell type or appearance for the site of collection (rule out spurious collection first).
- Uneven nuclear membrane thickening or clumping of chromatin along the nuclear membrane.
- Nuclear moulding.
- Cellular anaplasia (lack of differentiation).
- Cytoplasmic development uncoordinated with or inappropriate for the nuclear features.

FAQ24 How can I increase confidence in interpretation of malignancy and differentiation of malignant from nonmalignant features?

Confidence can be increased with experience and feedback. Features that help increase confidence in the presence of malignancy are:

- Large numbers of atypical cells that exhibit cytological criteria of malignancy.
- Monomorphic population of cells that is not complicated by a variety of cell types.
- Asymmetric mitotic figures.

It is harder to be confident if malignant cells are few, the overall cellularity is not high or if features of malignancy are subtle.

Comparison with the results of histology (if available) provides the best feedback. Correlation with clinical progression may be helpful in cases in which tissue confirmation is not available. Comparison with a report written by an experienced cytologist can also provide good feedback and an opportunity to learn.

With the advent of digital microscopic photography that can be transmitted via e-mail and the internet, it is possible to transmit images so that questions about particular cells or features can be analysed and information shared amongst cytologists. Although photographic images may not provide the same total picture as examination of the glass slide, they may provide valuable illustrations of significant features and may be very useful as a learning tool.

References

8

1. Freeman KP, Roszel JF, Slusher SH (1986) Patterns in equine endometrial cytologic smears. *Compendium on Continuing Education for the Practicing Veterinarian* **8**(7), 349–360.
2. Freeman KP, Roszel JF, Slusher SH, Kocan KM (1989) 'Repair cells' in equine uterine cytologic specimens. *Acta Cytologica* **33**(3), 397–402.

9

1. Schrank JH Jr, Dooley DP (1995) Purulent pericarditis caused by *Candida* species: case report and review. *Clinical Infectious Diseases* **21**(1), 182–187.
2. Baker R, Lumsden JH (2000) *Color Atlas of Cytology of the Dog and Cat* (1st edn). Mosby, St. Louis, pp. 23–29.

18

1. Sparkes AH, Gruffydd-Jones TJ, Harbour DA (1994) An appraisal of the value of laboratory tests in the diagnosis of feline infectious peritonitis. *Journal of the American Animal Hospital Association* **30**, 345–350.
2. Pedersen NC (1995) An overview of feline enteric coronavirus and feline infectious peritonitis. *Feline Practice* **23**(3), 7.

20

1. Freeman KP, Roszel JF (1997) Patterns in equine respiratory cytology specimens associated with respiratory conditions of noninfectious or unknown etiology. *Compendium on Continuing Education for the Practicing Veterinarian* **19**(6), 755–763, 783.
2. Freeman KP, Roszel JF (1997) Patterns in equine respiratory cytology specimens associated with respiratory conditions of known or suspected infectious etiology. *Compendium on Continuing Education for the Practicing Veterinarian* **19**(3), 378–383, 405.
3. Roszel JF, Freeman KP, Slusher SH *et al.* (1988) Siderophages in pulmonary cytology specimens from racing and nonracing horses. *Proceedings of the 33rd Convention of the American Association of Equine Practitioners*, New Orleans, pp. 321–329.
4. Step DL, Freeman KP, Gleed R, Hackett R (1991) Cytological and endoscopic findings after intrapulmonary blood inoculation in horses. *Journal of Equine Veterinary Science* **119**(6), 340–345.

23

Duesberg C, Petersen ME (1997) Adrenal disorders in cats. *Veterinary Clinics of North America (Small Animal)* **27**(2), 321–347.

26

1. Lagenbach A, McManus PM, Hendrick MJ *et al.* (2001) Sensitivity and specificity of methods of assessing the regional lymph nodes for evidence of metastasis in dogs and cats with solid tumors. *Journal of the American Veterinary Medical Association* **218**(9), 1424–1428.
2. Bankcroft JD, Stevens A (1996) (eds) *Theory and Practice of Histological Techniques* (4th edn). Churchill Livingston, Edinburgh.
3. Gross TL, Ihrke PJ, Walder J (1992) (eds) *Veterinary Dermatohistopathology: A Macroscopic and Microscopic Evaluation of Canine and Feline Skin Disease*. Mosby, St. Louis, p. 464.

32

1. Freeman KP, Roszel JF (1997) Patterns in equine respiratory cytology specimens associated with respiratory conditions of noninfectious or unknown etiology. *Compendium on Continuing Education for the Practicing Veterinarian* **19**(6), 755–763, 783.
2. Freeman KP, Roszel JF (1997) Patterns in equine respiratory cytology specimens associated with respiratory conditions of known or suspected infectious etiology. *Compendium on Continuing Education for the Practicing Veterinarian* **19**(3): 378–383, 405.
3. Roszel JF, Freeman KP, Slusher SH *et al.* (1988) Siderophages in pulmonary cytology specimens from racing and nonracing horses. *Proceedings of the 33rd Convention of the American Association of Equine Practitioners*, New Orleans, pp. 321–329.
4. Step DL, Freeman KP, Gleed R, Hackett R (1991) Cytological and endoscopic findings after intrapulmonary blood inoculation in horses. *Journal of Equine Veterinary Science* **119**(6), 340–345.

33

1. Lindsay DS, Blagburn BL, Dubey JP (1997) Feline toxoplasmosis and the importance of *Toxoplasma gondii* oocysts. *Compendium on Continuing Education for the Practicing Veterinarian* **19**(4), 448–461.
2. Lappin M (1999) Feline toxoplasmosis. *In Practice* **21**, 578–589.

35

1. Freeman KP, Carrol B (1989) Use of wet-fixed, trichrome-stained cytological specimens in private equine practice. *Compendium on Continuing Education for the Practicing Veterinarian* **11**(4), 485–494.

2. Freeman KP, Slusher SH, Roszel JF, Payne M (1986) Mycotic infections of the equine uterus. *Equine Practice* **8**(1), 34–42.
3. Freeman KP, Johnston JM (1987) Collaboration of a cytopathologist and equine practitioners using endometrial cytology in private broodmare practice. *Proceedings of the 33rd Convention of the American Association of Equine Practitioners*, New Orleans, pp. 629–639.
4. Roszel JF, Freeman KP (1988) Equine endometrial cytology. *Veterinary Clinics of North America (Equine)* **4**, 247–262.

38

1. Freeman KP, Slusher SH, Roszel JF, Payne M (1986) Mycotic infections of the equine uterus. *Equine Practice* **8**(1), 34–42.
2. Slusher SH, Freeman KP, Roszel JF (1985) Infertility diagnosis in mares using endometrial biopsy, culture and aspirate cytology. *Proceedings of the 31st Convention of the American Association of Equine Practitioners*, Toronto, p. 165.

52

1. Christopher M (1999) Pericardial fluid in a bearded dragon. Case review session No. 20. *The American Society for Veterinary Clinical Pathology*, Chicago.
2. Meyer DJ, Harvey JW (1999) *Veterinary Laboratory Medicine: Interpretation and Diagnosis* (2nd edn). WB Saunders, Philadelphia, p. 260.

65

1. Wright D, Bauman D (1999) *Georgis' Parasitology for Veterinarians* (7th edn). WB Saunders, Philadelphia, pp. 187–191.

References

2. Ettinger SJ, Feldman EC (1995) *Textbook of Veterinary Internal Medicine* (5th edn). WB Saunders, Philadelphia, pp. 1070–1071.
3. Fisher M (2001) Endoparasites in the dog and cat. *In Practice* **23**(8), 462–471.

66

Roth L (2001) Comparison of liver cytology and biopsy diagnosis in dogs and cats: 56 cases. *Veterinary Clinical Pathology* **30**(1), 35–38.

75

1. Gross TL, Ihrke PJ, Walder J (1992) (eds) *Veterinary Dermatohistopathology: A Macroscopic and Microscopic Evaluation of Canine and Feline Skin Disease*. Mosby, St. Louis, pp. 470–473.
2. Moulton JE (1978) (ed) *Tumors in Domestic Animals* (3rd edn). University of California Press, Berkeley, pp. 26–31.
3. Yager JA, Wilcock JP (1994) Tumors of the skin and associated tissues. In *Color Atlas and Text of Surgical Pathology of the Dog and Cat: Dermatopathology and Skin Tumors*. (eds JA Yager and JP Wilcock). Mosby, London, pp. 278–279.
4. Howard EB, Sawa TR, Nielsen SW, Kenyon AJ (1969) Mastocytoma and gastroduodenal ulceration. Gastric and duodenal ulcers in dogs with mastocytoma. *Veterinary Pathology* **6**(2), 146–158.
5. Rodgers KS (1993) Common questions about diagnosing and treating canine mast cell tumors. *Veterinary Medicine* **88**, 246–250.

97

Legendre AM (1995) Antimycotic drug therapy. In *Kirk's Current Veterinary Therapy XII* (ed JD Bonagura). WB Saunders, Philadelphia, pp. 327–331.

98

1. Freeman KP (1993) Cytologic evaluation of the equine mammary gland. Satellite article. *Equine Veterinary Education* **5**(4), 212–213.
2. Freeman KP, Slusher SH, Roszel JF, Young D (1988) Cytologic features of equine mammary secretions: normal and abnormal. *Compendium on Continuing Education for the Practicing Veterinarian* **10**(9), 1090–1100.

100

1. Cowell RL, Tyler RD, Meinkoth JH (1999) *Diagnostic Cytology and Hematology of the Dog and Cat* (2nd edn). Mosby, St. Louis, pp. 99–100.
2. Hsu SM, Hso PL, McMillan PN *et al.* (1982) Russell bodies: a light and electron microscopic immunoperoxidase study. *American Journal of Clinical Pathology* **77**, 26–31.

102

1. Meadows RL, MacWilliams PS (1994) Chylous effusions revisited. *Veterinary Clinical Pathology* **23**(2), 54–62.
2. Baker R, Lumsden JH (2000) *Color Atlas of Cytology of the Dog and Cat* (1st edn). Mosby, St. Louis, pp. 23–29.
3. Willard MD, Twedten H, Turnwald GH (1994) *Small Animal Clinical Diagnosis by Laboratory Methods* (2nd edn). WB Saunders, Philadelphia.

106

1. Moulton JE (1978) (ed) *Tumors in Domestic Animals* (3rd edn). University of California Press, Berkeley, pp. 36–38.
2. Gross TL, Ihrke PJ, Walder J (1992) (eds) *Veterinary Dermatohistopathology: A Macroscopic and Microscopic Evaluation of Canine and Feline Skin Disease*. Mosby, St. Louis, pp. 436–438.

3. Dernell WS, Withrow SJ, Kuntz CA, Powers BE (1998) Principles of treatment for soft tissue cell sarcoma. *Clinical Techniques in Small Animal Practice* **13(1)**, 59–64.

110

Walker AL, Jang SS, Hirsh DC (2000) Bacteria associated with pyothorax of dogs and cats: 98 cases (1989–1998). *Journal of the American Veterinary Medical Association* **216(3)**, 359–363.

112

1. Cotran RS, Kumar V, Collins T (1999) (eds) *Robbins Pathologic Basis of Disease* (6th edn). WB Saunders, Philadelphia, p. 196.
2. Baker R, Lumsden JH (2000) *Color Atlas of Cytology of the Dog and Cat* (1st edn). Mosby, St. Louis, pp. 23–29.
3. Feldman BF, Zinkl JG, Jain NC (2000) *Schalm's Veterinary Hematology* (5th edn). Lippincott Williams and Wilkins, Philadelphia, p. 304.
4. Jain NC (1993) *Essentials of Veterinary Hematology*. Lee & Febiger, Philadelphia, p. 253.

121

1. Roszel JF, Freeman KP (1988) Equine endometrial cytology. *Veterinary Clinics of North America (Equine)* **4(2)**, 247–262.
2. Slusher SH, Freeman KP, Roszel JF (1985) Infertility diagnosis in mares using endometrial biopsy, culture and aspirate cytology. *Proceedings of the 31st Convention of the American Association of Equine Practitioners*, Toronto, p. 165.
3. Freeman KP, Roszel JF, Slusher SH (1986) Patterns in equine endometrial cytologic smears. *Compendium on Continuing Education for the Practicing Veterinarian* **8(7)**, 349–360.

137

Borjesson LL, Christopher MM, Ling GV (1999) Detection of canine transitional cell carcinoma using a bladder tumor antigen dipstick test. *Veterinary Clinical Pathology* **28**, 33–38.

140

1. Hirschberger J, DeNicola DB, Hermanns W, Kraft W (1999) Sensitivity and specificity of cytologic evaluation in the diagnosis of neoplasia in body fluids from dogs and cats. *Veterinary Clinical Pathology* **28(4)**, 142–146.
2. Duncan JR, Prasse KW, Mahaffey EA (1994) *Veterinary Laboratory Medicine: Clinical Pathology* (3rd edn). Iowa State University Press, Ames, pp. 65–66.

141

1. Freeman KP, Roszel JF, Slusher SH (1986) Patterns in equine endometrial cytologic smears. *Compendium on Continuing Education for the Practicing Veterinarian* **8(7)**, 349–360.
2. Freeman KP, Johnston JM (1987) Collaboration of a cytopathologist and equine practitioners using endometrial cytology in private broodmare practice. *Proceedings of the 33rd Convention of the American Association of Equine Practitioners*, New Orelans, pp. 629–639.

148

1. Ettinger SJ, Feldman EC (1995) *Textbook of Veterinary Internal Medicine* (5th edn). WB Saunders, Philadelphia, pp. 1098–1099.
2. Cowel RL, Tyler RD, Meinkoth JH (1999) (eds) *Diagnostic Cytology and Hematology of the Dog and Cat* (2nd edn). Mosby, St. Louis, p. 182.

151

1. Shipstone M (2000) Generalised demodicosis in dogs: clinical perspective. *Australian Veterinary Journal* 78(**4**), 240–242.
2. Tamura Y, Kawamura Y, Inoue I, Ishino S (2001) Scanning electron microscopy description of a new species of *Demodex canis* spp. *Veterinary Dermatology* **12**, 275–278.
3. Desch CE, Hillier A (2003) *Demodex injai*: a new species of hair follicle mite (Acari: Demodecidae) from the domestic dog (Canidae). *Journal of Medical Entomology* **40**(**2**), 146–149.
4. Scott DW, Miller WH jnr, Griffin CE (2001) *Muller and Kirk's Small Animal Dermatology* (6th edn). WB Saunders, Philadelphia, p. 458.

152

1. Ettinger SJ, Feldman EC (1995) *Textbook of Veterinary Internal Medicine* (5th edn). WB Saunders, Philadelphia, pp. 1070–1071.
2. Scott DW (1980) External ear disorders. *Journal of the American Animal Hospital Association* **16**, 426–433.
3. Rausch FD, Skinner GW (1978) Incidence and treatment of budding yeast in canine otitis externa. *Modern Veterinary Practice* **53**, 914–915.

Additional reading

Raskin RE, Meyer DJ (2001) (eds) *Atlas of Canine and Feline Cytology*. WB Saunders, Philadelphia.

Harvey JW (2001) *Atlas of Veterinary Hematology: Blood and Bone Marrow of Domestic Animals*. WB Saunders, Philadelphia.

Campbell TW (1995) (ed) *Avian Hematology and Cytology* (2nd edn). Iowa State University Press, Ames.

Fournel-Fleury C, Magnol JP, Guelfi JF (1994) (eds) *Color Atlas of Cancer Cytology of the Dog and Cat*. Pratique Médicale et Chirurgicale de l'Animal de Compagnie, Paris.

Wellman ML, Radin MJ (1999) *Bone Marrow Evaluation in Dogs and Cats: Ralston Purina Clinical Handbook Series*. Gloyd Group, Wilmington, pp. 43–60.

Villiers E, Blackwood L (2005) (eds) *BSAVA Manual of Canine and Feline Clinical Pathology* (2nd edn). British Small Animal Veterinary Association, Gloucester.

Baker R, Lumsden JH (2000) (eds) *Color Atlas of Cytology of the Dog and Cat*. Mosby, St. Louis.

Cowell RL, Tyler RD, Meinkoth JH (1999) (eds) *Diagnostic Cytology and Hematology of the Dog and Cat* (2nd edn). Mosby, St. Louis.

Cowell RL, Tyler RD (2002) (eds) *Diagnostic Cytology and Hematology of the Horse* (2nd edn). Mosby, St. Louis.

Feldman BF, Zinkl JG, Jain NC (2000) *Schalm's Veterinary Hematology* (5th edn). Lippincott Williams & Wilkins, Philadelphia.

Thrall MA, Baker DC, Campbell TW, DeNicola D *et al.* (2004) *Veterinary Hematology and Clinical Chemistry*. Lippincott, Williams & Wilkins, Philadelphia.

Index